The Elbow in Sport
Injury, Treatment, and Rehabilitation

Todd S. Ellenbecker, MS, PT, SCS, CSCS
Physiotherapy Associates Scottsdale Sports Clinic

Angelo J. Mattalino, MD
Southwest Sports Medicine and Orthopaedic
Surgery Clinic, Ltd.

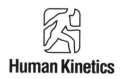

Human Kinetics

Library of Congress Cataloging-in-Publication Data

Ellenbecker, Todd S., 1962-
   The elbow in sport : injury, treatment, and rehabilitation / Todd
S. Ellenbecker, Angelo J. Mattalino.
     p.   cm.
   Includes bibliographical references and index.
   ISBN 0-87322-897-9
   1. Elbow--Wounds and injuries. 2. Sports injuries.
I. Mattalino, Angelo J., 1951- . II. Title.
   [DNLM: 1. Elbow--injuries. 2. Athletic Injuries. WE 820 E45e
1997]
RD558.E45   1997
617.5'74--dc 20
DNLM/DLC
  for Library of Congress   96-31956
                                              CIP

ISBN: 0-87322-897-9

Developmental Editor: Kirby Mittelmeier; **Assistant Editors:** Chad Johnson, Pam Johnson, Andrew Smith, and Sandra Merz Bott; **Editorial Assistant:** Amy Carnes; **Copyeditor:** Barbara Field; **Indexer:** Theresa Schaefer; **Graphic Designer:** Judy Henderson; **Graphic Artist:** Julie Overholt; **Photo Editor:** Boyd LaFoon; **Cover Designer:** Jack Davis; **Photographer (cover):** Anthony Neste; **Illustrator:** Beth Young; **Printer:** Braun-Brumfield

Printed in the United States of America   10 9 8 7 6 5 4 3 2 1

Human Kinetics
web site: http://www.humankinetics.com/

United States: Human Kinetics,
P.O. Box 5076
Champaign, IL 61825-5076
1-800-747-4457
e-mail: humank@hkusa.com

Canada: Human Kinetics,
Box 24040, Windsor, ON N8Y 4Y9
1-800-465-7301 (in Canada only)
e-mail: humank@hkcanada.com

Europe: Human Kinetics,
P.O. Box IW14, Leeds LS16 6TR
United Kingdom

(44) 1132 781708
email: humank@hkeurope.com

Australia: Human Kinetics
57A Price Avenue
Lower Mitcham
South Australia 5062
(08) 277 1555
e-mail: humank@hkaustralia.com

New Zealand: Human Kinetics,
P.O. Box 105-231, Auckland 1
(09) 523 3462
e-mail: humank@hknewz.com

To my wife, Gail, for her constant support, encouragement, and patience,
to my father and mother for their lifelong guidance,
and to George Davies, Janet Sobel, and Gary Derscheid
for their tremendous gifts of mentorship.

TSE

Contents

Preface

Most sport-related injuries to the elbow are overuse in nature and respond favorably to a nonoperative treatment plan that is part of a total arm strength rehabilitation program. The purpose of this book is to provide rehabilitation professionals—physical therapists, athletic trainers, strength and conditioning professionals, and sport scientists—the rationale and background for treating and rehabilitating overuse injuries in the athletic elbow.

The inherent design of the elbow joint and its vulnerability to overuse injury in sports make evaluation and treatment of this joint a clinical challenge. Furthermore, the elbow's interdependence with the upper extremity kinetic chain necessitates a total extremity or total arm strength approach in both evaluation and treatment. The book's early emphasis on the anatomy and biomechanics of the elbow, including kinetic and kinematic analysis of the elbow in sport-specific activities, is meant to provide the framework for a comprehensive evaluation and total arm treatment approach. Detailed descriptions of approaches to nonoperative injury management illustrate how resistive exercise, range of motion, and biomechanical analysis are applied to rehabilitate the athletic elbow, while surgical descriptions and explanation of specific diagnostic tests and imaging techniques enhance postoperative understanding for clinicians, increasing their understanding of patient symptoms following surgical procedures.

To help provide an objective rationale for the methods used in treating this population, clinical research on musculoskeletal adaptations and range of motion and strength of the distal upper extremity kinetic chain is included. Finally, actual case studies are included to help synthesize the rehabilitative concepts discussed throughout the book.

Acknowledgments

The authors would like to thank several individuals who have assisted with this book: Rich Boeckmann, PT, Jeff Kitchen, PT, and David Schulz, PT, for their editorial assistance; Veronica Serna, ATC, for her illustrations; and Gail Haertel, MS, and Carlyn Hakola for their technical assistance.

Introduction

The repetitive physiological and mechanical stresses imparted to the elbow during activities of daily living (ADL), especially those involving overhead sport activities such as the throwing motion or the tennis serve, can cause specific and characteristic overuse injuries to the joint. Many of the published reports on overuse elbow injury focus on the throwing or overhead motion athlete.

In a review of 100 consecutive records of symptomatic baseball pitchers, Barnes and Tullos (1978) found a 50 percent incidence of elbow injury. Tullos and King (1973) report that 50 percent of professional baseball pitchers experience elbow or shoulder symptoms at some point in their careers that do not allow them to continue pitching. Table 1 presents a review of

TABLE 1 Epidemiology of Overuse Elbow Injury in Upper-Extremity-Dominant Sports

Population	Age (yrs)	Sample size	Incidence (%)	Reference
Professional baseball players	—	100	50	Barnes & Tullos, 1978
Female collegiate softball pitchers	17-23	24	8	Loosli et al., 1992
Tennis players:				
Elite juniors	14-17	32	12	USTA, unpublished data
Danish elite professionals	14-18	104	11	Winge et al., 1989
Recreational	Adults	231	47	Priest et al., 1977
Recreational	Adults	534	38	Hang & Peng, 1984
Recreational	Adults	—	50	Kamien, 1990
Recreational	Adults	150	41	Kitai et al., 1986
Recreational	Adults	77	35	Carroll, 1981

epidemiological studies of athletes that use the upper extremity extensively. A high incidence of overuse elbow injury is clearly evident in these populations.

Additionally, Adams (1968) reported a 95 percent incidence of elbow and shoulder injuries in 80 little league pitchers, the most common being accelerated growth and separation of the medial epicondylar epiphysis. Although Torg et al. (1972) reported less serious injuries in 49 preadolescent pitchers, shoulder or elbow soreness while throwing was reported by 70 percent of the subjects. The demands placed on the elbow of the immature athlete also result in overuse injury, often with specific osseous complications (Adams, 1968; Torg et al., 1972).

A further review of the epidemiological literature provides reinforcement for an important clinical evaluation and treatment principle discussed in this book called the "total arm strength" rehabilitation principle. This principle involves the use of evaluative and rehabilitative procedures for the *entire upper extremity kinetic chain*, not merely for the localized structures about the elbow itself. The clinical application and further-research-oriented rationale for the total arm strength approach to rehabilitation is incorporated into the treatment and evaluation portions of this text.

In a survey of 84 world-class tennis players, Priest and Nagel (1976) reported that 74 percent of men and 60 percent of women had a history of shoulder or elbow injury on the dominant arm that affected tennis play. Injuries to both the shoulder and elbow were reported by 21 and 23 percent of the men and women, respectively. The close interplay between the shoulder and elbow in the upper extremity kinetic chain is further demonstrated in a later study by Priest, Braden, and Gerberich (1980). In a survey of 2633 recreational tennis players, a 31 percent incidence of tennis elbow was reported. An additional finding in this study, however, was the 63 percent greater incidence of shoulder injury among those players reporting a history of humeral epicondylitis.

Classifying Injuries to the Elbow

Overuse injuries to the athletic elbow occur from the repetitive stresses inherent in upper extremity movements. Although traumatic injuries to the elbow such as fractures and dislocations do occur in sport activities, they are beyond the scope of this text. The most commonly reported overuse injuries to the elbow are

- humeral (lateral and medial) epicondylitis,
- ulnar collateral ligament injury,
- ulnar nerve dysfunction (neuritis),

- osteochondral injury (osteophytes/loose bodies), and
- growth plate injury (in adolescents).

Further classification of elbow injuries incurred with throwing include medial tension, or tensile overload, and lateral compression (Barnes & Tullos, 1978; Bennett, 1959; Slocum, 1978). Attenuation of the ulnar collateral ligament and ulnar nerve as well as medial epicondylar growth plate injury are examples of medial tension injuries, and osteochondral lesions of the radial head is a prime example of a lateral compression injury.

Andrews (Joyce, Jelsma, & Andrews, 1995) has further refined the original classification of medial tension and lateral compression set up by Bennett and Slocum into a broad category termed valgus extension overload. The combined valgus and forceful elbow extension stresses placed on the joint during the acceleration phase of throwing lead to characteristic injury to the ulnar collateral ligament and posteromedial bony structures of the elbow. The etiology of each of these overuse injuries will be detailed later in this book.

CHAPTER 1

Anatomy and Biomechanics of the Elbow

Extensive knowledge of upper extremity kinetic chain anatomy and analysis of muscular activity patterns, joint kinetics, and kinematics of the elbow during characteristic upper extremity sport activities provide the framework for a better understanding of elbow injury etiology and allow for more comprehensive evaluation and clinical treatment of overuse injuries in the athletic elbow. A thorough grasp of this information also allows the clinician to prepare the injured areas more specifically for a functional return to the inherent demands of the sport activity that produced the injury. Finally, analyzing the relationship between faulty biomechanical execution of upper extremity movement patterns and elbow injury is a major part of the total rehabilitative effort in the athlete with an overuse elbow injury.

Arthrology/Osteology

The elbow is technically termed a trochoginglymoid joint (Morrey, 1993). It is composed of three individual joints—the ulnohumeral, radiohumeral, and proximal radioulnar—all enclosed in one joint capsule. The ulnohumeral joint provides the primary hinge-type motion of flexion/extension, with the radiohumeral and proximal radioulnar joints providing the rotational or pivoting motions of pronation/supination.

The distal humerus consists of two condyles forming the articular surfaces of the trochlea and capitellum. Just proximal to the trochlea is the medial epicondyle, which is more prominent than the lateral epicondyle and serves as the attachment for the flexor-pronator muscle group and ulnar collateral ligament.

The distal humerus is internally rotated 3° to 8° with respect to a line joining the epicondyles when viewed from the axial plane (figure 1.1a). The trochlea is an hourglass-shaped projection that articulates with the semilunar notch of the proximal ulna. The trochlea has a continuous arch of cartilage of 300° to 330° distally, allowing for smooth interface with the proximal ulna (Morrey, 1993). The medial aspect of the trochlea is larger and projects farther distally, resulting in an overall valgus tilt in the frontal plane of 6° with respect to the long axis of the humerus (figure 1.1b) (Stroyan & Wilk, 1993). This distal projection of the medial aspect of the trochlea, termed the carrying angle, results in a normal valgus angulation of the elbow.

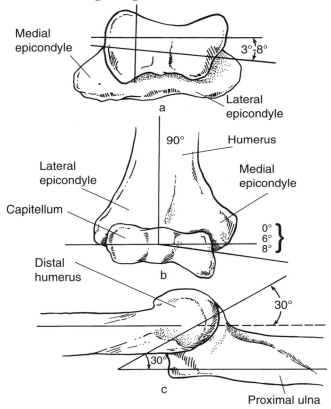

FIGURE 1.1 Angular relationships of the distal humerus: (a) inferior view of the distal humerus showing 3° to 8° of internal rotation of the distal humerus with respect to a line joining the medial and lateral epicondyles; (b) anterior view of the distal humerus showing 6° to 8° of valgus tilt with respect to the long axis; and (c) side view of the ulnohumeral joint demonstrating the 30° posterior angulation of the sigmoid notch and 30° anterior tilt of the distal humerus allowing full extension of the elbow.

The ulnohumeral joint has very congruent surfaces and is responsible for up to 50 percent of the varus/valgus stability of the elbow joint (Jobe & Kvitne, 1991). The distal humerus is oriented 30° anterior to the long axis of the humerus in the sagittal plane, with a corresponding 30° posterior angulation of the greater sigmoid notch of the proximal ulna that receives the trochlea (figure 1.1c). This angular arrangement allows for full elbow extension and 140° to 150° of elbow flexion without abutment of the bony surfaces.

The distal humerus has three depressions, or fossae, that further allow full range of motion. Anteriorly, the coronoid fossa lies just proximal to the trochlea and receives the coronoid process of the ulna (figure 1.2). The radial fossa is just proximal to the capitellum and creates a depression for the radial head during full flexion. Posteriorly, the olecranon fossa receives the olecranon process during extension of the ulnohumeral joint.

Lateral to the coronoid of the ulna is the lesser sigmoid fossa, which articulates with the head of the radius. The lesser sigmoid fossa forms an arc of approximately 60° to 80°, which results in an excursion of 180° of pronation/supination range of motion. The proximal aspect of the radius contains a concave depression termed the radial head, which is not totally cylindrical but slightly oval (Stroyan & Wilk, 1993). The head and neck of the radius are not collinear but form an angle of 15° with respect to the shaft of the radius (Morrey, 1993; Stroyan & Wilk, 1993).

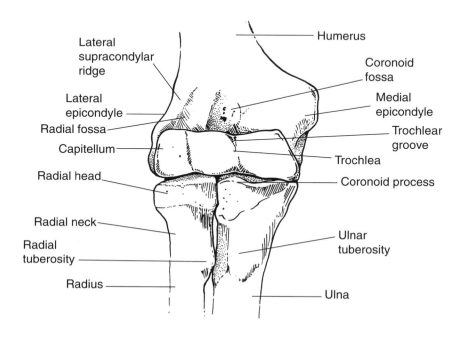

FIGURE 1.2   The bony landmarks of the elbow (anterior view).

Capsuloligamentous Structures

The osseous relationships outlined above clearly demonstrate the intricate articular relationships that form the elbow joint as well as the high degree of bony congruity compared to the more proximal glenohumeral joint. In addition to the static stability provided by the articular geometry, ligamentous structures about the elbow also play an integral role in maintaining joint stability.

Capsule

The capsule of the elbow (shown with major neural structures in figure 1.3) follows the perimeter of the elbow and distally blends with the annular ligament. The anterior aspect of the capsule becomes taut with the elbow in the extended position and provides a stabilizing effect via thickenings within its structure (Morrey, 1993). The posterior aspect of the joint capsule becomes taut with elbow flexion. The capsule includes all three joints as well as the radial, coronoid, and olecranon fossae.

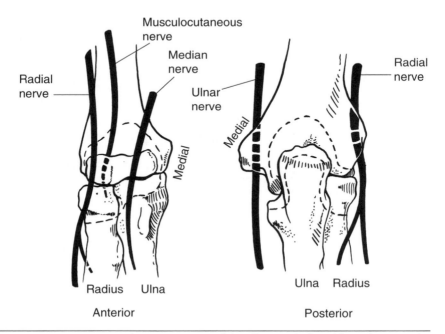

FIGURE 1.3   Anterior and posterior views of the elbow with dotted lines depicting the margins of the elbow joint capsule.

Medial (Ulnar) Collateral Ligament

The ulnar or medial collateral ligament (MCL) comprises three specific sections on the medial aspect of the ulnohumeral joint (figure 1.4). The MCL originates from the entire inferior aspect of the medial epicondyle. The humeral origin of the anterior band (or bundle) is eccentrically located with respect to the axis of elbow extension and flexion and thus provides stability throughout these ranges of motion (Jobe & Kvitne, 1991).

The anterior band inserts into the anteromedial portion of the coronoid of the ulna. This insertion site gives the anterior band a significant mechanical advantage in controlling valgus forces. The anterior band of the ulnar collateral ligament consists of distinct collagen bundles within the layers of the capsule, with an additional ligament complex superficial to the capsular layers (Timmerman & Andrews, 1994b). Only the anterior 20 to 30 percent of the ulnar collateral ligament is visible from the anterior portal during arthroscopy (Timmerman & Andrews, 1994b). The posterior band of the ulnar collateral ligament originates posterior and inferior to the axis of rotation and inserts into the medial aspect of the semilunar notch of the proximal ulna. Due to the orientation of the posterior band, it becomes taut after 60° (Morrey & An, 1983) to 90° (Jobe & Kvitne, 1991) of elbow flexion. The posterior band of the ulnar collateral ligament consists of distinct collagen bundles within the capsular layers, with 30 to 50 percent of the posterior aspect visible through the posterior arthroscopic portal. The transverse band does not cross the joint but acts as a thickening of the caudal-most portion of the joint capsule to expand the semilunar (sigmoid) notch and, according to most sources, does not contribute to joint stability (Jobe & Kvitne, 1991; Morrey & An, 1983; Stroyan & Wilk, 1993).

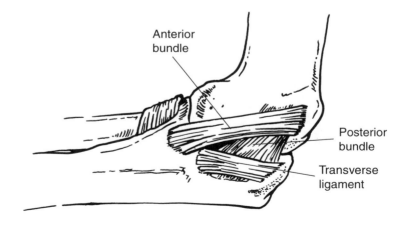

FIGURE 1.4   Medial collateral ligament complex.

The ulnar nerve rests in the posterior aspect of the medial epicondyle but is not intimately related to the fibers of the ulnar collateral ligament (Morrey & An, 1983).

Lateral Ligamentous Structures

The lateral ligament complex of the elbow is less defined and more variable than the medial (ulnar) collateral ligament. The lateral ligament complex consists of the radial collateral ligament, lateral ulnar collateral ligament, accessory lateral collateral ligament, and annular ligament (figure 1.5).

The lateral or radial collateral ligament originates from the lateral epicondyle and is less defined than the ulnar collateral ligament. It inserts into the annular ligament and provides an area of origin for a portion of the supinator muscle (Morrey, 1993). Due to the close approximation of the origin of the radial collateral ligament to the center of rotation of the elbow joint, this ligament remains taut throughout the range of elbow extension and flexion and provides both stability to varus stress and approximation of the radiocapitellar joint (King, Morrey, & An, 1993).

The lateral ulnar collateral ligament spans the radiocapitellar joint, superficial to the annular ligament, and inserts onto the crista musculi supinatoris. This portion of the lateral ligament complex provides stability to resist varus stress of the elbow. O'Driscoll, Bell, and Morrey (1991) report posterolateral rotary instability of the ulnohumeral joint with release of the lateral ulnar collateral ligament. They consider the lateral ulnar col-

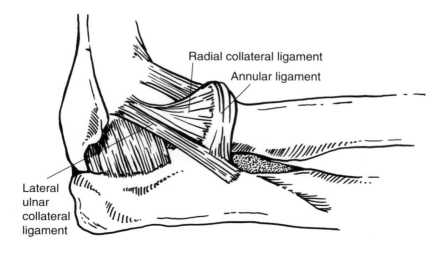

FIGURE 1.5   Lateral collateral ligament complex.

lateral ligament, which is taut in both extension and flexion, to be the primary lateral stabilizer of the elbow. Sojbjerg, Ovesen, and Nielsen (1987) studied the lateral collateral ligament complex and reported only a minor influence on varus stability. It is suggested that its main role is prevention of distal migration of the annular ligament.

The accessory lateral collateral ligament originates from the inferior margin of the annular ligament and inserts into the tubercle of the supinator crest. Its function is to further stabilize the annular ligament during varus stress (Morrey, 1993).

The annular ligament is a fibro-osseous ring that stabilizes the radial head. It originates and inserts on the anterior and posterior margins of the lesser sigmoid notch. With supination of the forearm, the anterior aspect of the ligament becomes taut, whereas pronation of the forearm causes tension in the posterior aspect.

Finally, the oblique cord and quadrate ligament are additional ligamentous structures that lend only minor stabilizing influence to the elbow joint. Both structures are reported to have minimal functional significance (Stroyan & Wilk, 1993).

Ligaments and Elbow Stability

Stability of the elbow is provided by a combination of the articular geometry and capsuloligamentous structures. Table 1.1, from An and Morrey (1993), shows the relative contribution of the capsule, bony articulations, and ligaments to rotational or distraction force. Of particular importance is the change in contribution to valgus force of the MCL relative to the bony articulation and joint capsule between the extended and flexed positions. In the extended position, the bony articulation provides 31 percent of the restraining force to valgus stress, as does the MCL. With the elbow in the flexed position, however, the bony articulation accounts for 33 percent of the restraining force, with 54 percent now coming from the MCL. Additionally, the capsule accounts for 38 percent of the restraining force to valgus stress in elbow extension but only 10 percent in flexion, placing even greater relative responsibility on the MCL.

This detailed analysis of the relative contributions to elbow stability highlights the vulnerability of the joint and its reliance on the MCL to deter valgus stresses, especially with the elbow in a flexed position. Biomechanical analysis of the throwing motion and tennis serve demonstrates high valgus stresses to the medial elbow occurring during the acceleration phase with the elbow in a position of approximately 90° of flexion (Kibler, 1994; Werner, Fleisig, Dillman, & Andrews, 1993). The incidence of injury from valgus stresses applied to the elbow is explained by these anatomical analyses.

TABLE 1.1   Percent Contribution of Restraining Force During Displacement (Rotational or Distractional)

Position	Stabilizing element	Distraction	Varus	Valgus
Extension	MCL	12	—	31
	LCL	10	14	—
	Capsule	70	32	38
	Articulation	—	55	31
Flexion	MCL	78	—	54
	LCL	10	9	—
	Capsule	8	13	10
	Articulation	—	75	33

MCL = Medial collateral ligament complex; LCL = Lateral collateral ligament complex

Data from Morrey 1993.

Neural Anatomy

A basic outline of the proximal and distal course of the major neural structures about the elbow enables the clinician to better appreciate the local injury often present in the athletic elbow. A more specific, detailed description of the neural structures of the elbow will be given in the discussion of specific overuse pathology later in this book. Figure 1.3 shows the relationship of the major neural structures to the elbow joint.

Median Nerve

The median nerve arises from branches off the lateral and medial cords of the brachial plexus and is composed of nerve root levels C5-8 and T1. As the nerve proceeds distally over the anterior aspect of the brachium, passing beneath the brachial fascia and anterior to the brachialis muscle, it continues on a relatively straight course to the medial aspect of the antecubital fossa just medial to both the biceps tendon and brachial artery. The median nerve passes under the bicipital aponeurosis (lacertus fibrosis) and through the two heads of the pronator teres muscle before giving off a branch called the anterior interosseous nerve at the inferior aspect of the pronator teres; this branch continues along the anterior aspect of the interosseous membrane. The median nerve can be compressed between the two heads of the pronator teres, due to forceful repetitive pronatory movements, as well as under the bicipital aponeurosis (Morrey, 1993; Stroyan & Wilk, 1993).

Radial Nerve

The radial nerve is the largest branch of the brachial plexus, arising as a continuation of the posterior cord from the C6, C7, and C8 levels, with variable involvement of the C5 and T1 levels. As the nerve progresses distally, it descends through the radial groove of the humerus near the midportion of the brachium and continues laterally to penetrate the intermuscular septum. The nerve descends anterior to the lateral epicondyle, and posterior to the brachialis and brachioradialis muscles, before splitting at the level of the radiocapitellar joint into the posterior interosseous (motor) and superficial radial (sensory) branches. The superficial radial branch continues distally to lie under the brachioradialis and anterior to the pronator teres and supinator muscles. The posterior interosseous branch curves around the posterior lateral aspect of the radius and passes between the two heads of the supinator. This is significant due to the presence of a fibrous arch, called the arcade of Frohse, near the proximal edge of the supinator muscle in approximately 30 percent of the population. Entrapment of the posterior interosseous nerve can occur with forceful, repetitive supination or pronation movements.

Musculocutaneous Nerve

This nerve originates from the lateral cord of the brachial plexus and is composed of nerve root levels C5-7. The nerve passes between the biceps and brachialis muscles to pierce the brachial fascia lateral to the biceps tendon and continues on to terminate as the lateral antebrachial cutaneous nerve.

Ulnar Nerve

The ulnar nerve is formed from the medial cord of the brachial plexus (C8 and T1) and courses distally in the medial intermuscular septum in a posterior position along the medial margin of the triceps. The nerve passes through the arcade of Struthers, a fascial structure bridging the medial head of the triceps and the intermuscular septum, which is located approximately 8 cm proximal to the medial epicondyle. The ulnar nerve passes into the cubital tunnel beneath the medial epicondyle, resting against the ulnar collateral ligament via a groove within that structure (Morrey, 1993), and undergoes compression as it courses around and under the medial epicondyle.

The ulnar nerve is contained by a structure that forms the roof of the tunnel termed the cubital tunnel retinaculum by Morrey (figure 1.6). This structure originates on the medial epicondyle and crosses over the cubital groove to insert on the olecranon and triceps fascia. Flexion of the elbow tenses the cubital tunnel retinaculum and causes a flattening effect, placing greater pressure on the ulnar nerve compared to the elbow extension position, which relaxes this structure. The flattening of the cubital tunnel retinaculum during flexion of the elbow is of further consequence to the ulnar nerve in the presence of bony encroachment from osteophyte formation in the cubital groove region. This will be discussed extensively in chapter 2. Absence of the cubital tunnel retinaculum leads to congenital subluxation of the ulnar nerve and can lead to ulnar nerve pathology from friction and external irritation due to the hypermobility of the nerve and its close association with the surrounding structures (Morrey, 1993).

The ulnar nerve enters the forearm by passing between the two heads of the flexor carpi ulnaris. Aggressive flexion and ulnar deviation of the wrist can cause compression of the ulnar nerve as it passes between the two heads of the flexor carpi ulnaris.

Cutaneous Innervation

The cutaneous innervation of the elbow is supplied by five sensory nerves derived from four nerve root levels: C5, C6, T1, and T2. The approximate distribution of sensory innervation both anteriorly and posteriorly is found in figure 1.7.

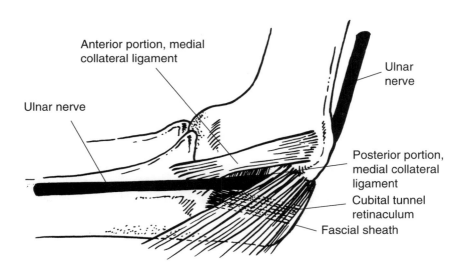

FIGURE 1.6 Medial view of the elbow depicting the course of the ulnar nerve and stabilizing influence of the cubital tunnel retinaculum (CTR).

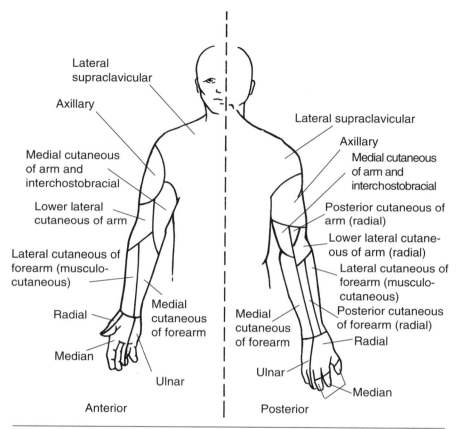

FIGURE 1.7   Cutaneous sensation distribution of the upper extremity.

Muscles

Functionally, the muscles about the elbow can be grouped as elbow extensors, elbow flexors, wrist flexors/forearm pronators, and wrist extensors/forearm supinators.

An, Hui, Morrey, Linscheid, and Chao (1981) studied the muscular structures around the elbow extensively and through moment arm analysis found that, although a majority of the muscles create moments about all three axes, most have only one dominant principal axis.

The muscles with the greatest moment arm in elbow flexion are the brachioradialis, biceps, brachialis, and extensor carpi radialis. The muscles with the greatest moment arms in elbow extension are the triceps, flexor carpi ulnaris, and anconeus. The flexor carpi radialis muscle was found to have an extension moment arm with the elbow in the extended position, but it changed to provide a flexion moment arm as the elbow became flexed (An et al., 1981). Muscles creating a valgus moment arm relative to the elbow joint center at the trochlea were the anconeus, brachioradialis, extensor carpi radialis, and extensor carpi ulnaris. The pronator teres, flexor carpi radialis, and flexor carpi ulnaris all created varus moments about the elbow and would resist valgus stress at the elbow. The moment arm data for the musculature surrounding the elbow indicate the efficiency of the muscle for rotation about a particular axis and provide a detailed rationale for specific, scientifically oriented muscular strengthening during rehabilitation of the athletic elbow.

The detailed anatomical descriptions of the primary muscles involved in overuse injury will be discussed in the section describing each injury later in this book. Table 1.2 serves as a resource, listing the muscles by function with their respective motor innervation.

In addition to a detailed understanding of the anatomical structures in the elbow, optimal treatment and understanding of the athlete with an overuse elbow injury requires a thorough understanding of the biomechanics of the elbow.

Muscular Activity Patterns

Indwelling electromyographic (EMG) analysis of muscles that cross the elbow and forearm effectively demonstrates structures at risk for injury as well as muscles that require additional strength, power, and endurance to enhance performance and prevent injury. To better understand the demands placed on the elbow joint, the throwing motion and tennis serve will be discussed, as well as tennis groundstrokes (forehand and backhand) and the golf swing. This review of muscular activity patterns highlights the predominant and consistent activity of the wrist and forearm musculature. Analyzing these muscular activity patterns helps explain the pattern of injury developed with sport-specific movement patterns.

Throwing Motion and Tennis Serve

The throwing (pitching) motion in baseball and the tennis serve are usually divided into four phases: windup, cocking, acceleration, and follow-through (Glousman, Barron, Jobe, Perry, & Pink, 1992; Morris, Jobe, Perry, Pink, & Healy, 1989; Werner et al., 1993). Sisto et al. (1987) and Glousman et al. (1992) studied the muscular activity patterns of the elbow musculature during the fastball pitch, and Morris et al. (1989) studied the muscular activity patterns during the tennis serve. Data from their studies are shown in table 1.3. Muscular activity during EMG analysis is measured as a percentage of the baseline activity during a maximal-intensity manual muscle

TABLE 1.2 Muscles of the Elbow and Forearm and Their Respective Motor Innervation

	Muscle/action	Innervation
Elbow flexors		
	Biceps brachii	(C5,6)
	Brachialis	(C5,6)
	Brachioradialis	(C5,6)
	Supinator	(C5,6,7)
Elbow extensors		
	Triceps brachii	(C6,7,8,T1)
	Anconeus	(C7,8)
Forearm pronators		
	Pronator teres	(C6,7)
	Pronator quadratus	(C7,8,T1)
	Flexor carpi radialis	(C5,6,7,8)
Forearm supinators		
	Biceps brachii	(C5,6)
	Supinator	(C5,6,7)
	Brachioradialis	(C5,6)
Wrist flexors		
	Flexor carpi radialis	(C6,7,8)
	Flexor carpi ulnaris	(C7,8,T1)
	Palmaris longus	(C7,8,T1)
	Flexor digitorum superficialis	(C7,8,T1)
	Flexor digitorum profundus	(C7,8,T1)
	Flexor pollicis longus	(C6,7,8,T1)
Wrist extensors		
	Extensor carpi radialis longus	(C5,6,7,8)
	Extensor carpi radialis brevis	(C5,6,7,8)
	Extensor carpi ulnaris	(C6,7,8)
	Extensor digitorum	(C6,7,8)
	Extensor digiti minimi	(C6,7,8)
	Extensor indicis	(C6,7,8)
	Extensor pollicis longus	(C6,7,8)

test (MMT). Values expressed in table 1.3 represent the level of muscular activity during each phase of the activity relative to this MMT. The baseball pitch and tennis serve will be discussed together in this section to compare the muscular activity patterns of these two overhead sport activities.

The windup phase of the pitching motion in baseball terminates when the dominant hand and ball leave the glove and the front leg begins to stride toward home plate. The six muscles tested had minimal activity during the windup phase of the throwing motion. During this phase, the forearm is slightly pronated, whereas the wrist is in slight extension.

TABLE 1.3 Muscular Activity Patterns of the Distal Upper Extremity During Throwing Motion (Pitch) and Tennis Serve*

	Muscle	Windup	Cocking		Acceleration		Follow-through	
Pitch	Biceps	—	22	26	25	—	27	—
Serve		9	7	11	12	14		34
Pitch	Triceps	—	17	37	89	—	42	—
Serve		5	2	36	65	20		9
Pitch	Pronator	—	18	39	85	—	34	—
Serve	teres	8	8	14	67	18		14
Pitch	FCR	—	24	47	120	—	60	—
Serve		5	9	24	41	25		11
Pitch	ECRL	—	53	72	30	—	29	—
Serve		22	17	63	31	29		18
Pitch	ECRB	—	46	75	55	—	37	—
Serve		17	33	70	49	21		25

ECRB = Extensor carpi radialis brevis, ECRL = Extensor carpi radialis longus, FCR = Flexor carpi radialis
*Values expressed as percentage of maximal manual muscle test (MMT).

The early cocking phase begins as the ball is released from the glove and continues until the front foot contacts the ground. The late cocking phase begins with front foot contact and terminates with maximal external rotation of the dominant shoulder. The elbow is flexed during this phase, with wrist and metacarpophalangeal joint extension activity predominating. Muscular activity is at peak levels in the wrist extensors. Moderate activity is found in the brachioradialis and pronator teres when a fastball is thrown. Shortly before the shoulder reaches maximal external rotation, the elbow extends slightly. During late cocking, the elbow is positioned in approximately 90° of flexion (Fleisig, Dillman, & Andrews, 1989) with forearm pronation and continued wrist extension.

The acceleration phase of the pitching motion begins following maximal external rotation of the dominant shoulder and ends at ball release (Fleisig et al., 1989). During the acceleration phase, the elbow is violently extended from 89° to 20° (Feltner & Dapena, 1986), resulting in peak muscular activity levels in the flexor carpi radialis, pronator teres, and triceps muscles. Some of the elbow extension force is contributed to centrifugal force generated by shoulder rotation. Evidence of the role of proximal body contribution to elbow extension force comes from a study by Roberts, which demonstrated subjects' ability to throw at 80 percent of maximal velocity with paralyzation of the triceps muscle on the dominant arm (Werner et al., 1993).

The follow-through phase begins with termination of the acceleration phase at ball release. Maximal pronation of the forearm and internal rotation of the humerus occurs during follow-through. Deceleration of the elbow is achieved through eccentric contraction of the biceps muscle. This eccentric deceleration is imperative to ensure controlled achievement of elbow extension range of motion during the throwing motion. Muscular activity in the triceps, anconeus, and wrist flexors also helps the joint ligaments apply a compression force and prevent elbow distraction (Werner et al., 1993).

The difference in muscular activity levels between a fastball and curve is most evident during the late cocking and acceleration phases. With the curveball, significantly greater wrist extensor activity was found in late cocking and especially acceleration, and continuing on into follow-through, suggesting a modified or altered hand and wrist position necessary for proper execution (Perry & Glousman, 1990). Sakurai, Ikegami, Okamoto, Yabe, and Toyoshima (1993) also report an alteration in the hand position during the late cocking phase of throwing a curveball. The forearm is held in more degrees of supination and slightly less wrist extension for a curveball compared to a fastball (Sakarai et al., 1993).

With the exception of the windup, all phases of the throwing motion require moderate to high levels of muscular activation. Optimal strength and endurance of these muscles is of key importance to protect the osseous and capsuloligamentous structures of the elbow. Evidence of the important role played by the elbow musculature is found in an EMG study by Glousman et al. (1992) comparing muscle activity in normal pitchers to those with ulnar collateral ligament injury. Greater activation of the extensor carpi radialis longus and brevis muscles was found in the ligamentously injured population, as well as significantly less flexor carpi radialis, pronator teres, and triceps activity.

Changes in muscle activation occurred only during the late cocking and follow-through phases of both the fastball and curveball pitches. The asynchronous firing pattern of the flexor and pronator muscle groups in the MCL-deficient pitchers demonstrates the possibility of further injuring the medial or lateral aspect of the elbow due to loss of necessary muscular stabilization. The increase in wrist extensor activity is relatively unexplained by the authors but may be due to a compensatory mechanism to protect the medial ligamentous structures. Finally, greater brachioradialis muscle activation was found in the injured elbows. This may be due to the greater degree of pronation found in the injured pitchers' delivery, giving this muscle greater mechanical advantage to function as a decelerator to protect the joint from end-range extension and protect the MCL.

The windup phase of the tennis serve terminates when the ball is released by the contralateral extremity. Consistent with EMG analysis of the throwing motion, the tennis serve has minimal muscular activity during the windup phase.

The cocking phase begins as the ball is tossed and ends at the point of maximal external rotation of the dominant shoulder (Morris et al., 1989).

Most of the muscular activity in the cocking phase is found in the biceps and the extensor carpi radialis brevis (ECRB) and extensor digitorum communis (wrist and finger extensors).

The acceleration phase of the tennis serve begins following maximal external rotation of the dominant arm and ends at ball impact. The predominant distal muscular activity occurs in the pronator teres, flexor carpi radialis, ECRB, triceps, and biceps (Morris et al., 1989). The biceps again plays a vital role in eccentrically decelerating the elbow to prevent excessive end-range elbow extension.

The follow-through phase is not characterized by extremely high levels of activity in the muscles crossing the elbow, forearm, and wrist. The biceps is again active during this phase as a decelerator of elbow extension and forearm pronation. All other muscles in the distal extremity are classified as low activity (<25 percent MMT) during this phase.

A relatively consistent pattern of muscular activity is reported to occur in skilled tennis players (Groppel & Nirschl, 1986; Miyashita, Tsunoda, Sakurai, Nishizono, & Mizuno, 1980; Yoshizawa, Itani, & Jonsson, 1987). The presence of increased as well as overlapping muscular activity patterns across the outlined stages has been reported in untrained and less-skilled tennis players. Increased muscular activity and asynchronous firing patterns highlight the inefficiency of the kinetic chain principle (see chapter 5) and a greater reliance on distal muscular activity for force generation rather than proper use of the lower extremities and trunk (Groppel & Nirschl, 1986).

Tennis Groundstrokes

The forehand and backhand groundstrokes in tennis can be broken down into three phases: preparation, acceleration, and follow-through (table 1.4) (Groppel & Nirschl, 1986; Rhu et al., 1988). To define these stages for research, the preparation phase begins with the first motion of the racquet and arm during the backswing and ends with the first forward motion of the racquet. Muscular activity is very low during the preparation phase of both the forehand and backhand, with the exception of the wrist extensors on the forehand (Morris et al., 1989).

The acceleration phase begins with the forward movement of the racquet and arm and ends with ball contact. During the acceleration phase of the forehand, very high wrist extensor activation is present, with a very low level in the pronator teres and wrist flexors (Morris et al., 1989). The extensor carpi radialis brevis and longus, extensor communis, and biceps and brachioradialis all exhibit high levels of muscular activity during this phase of the forehand groundstroke. Contrary to popular belief, vigorous topspin during the acceleration phase of the forehand is not produced by hyperpronation of the forearm. This is confirmed in the EMG analysis of tennis groundstrokes (table 1.4) (Groppel & Nirschl, 1986).

The acceleration phase of the backhand groundstroke consists of high activity in the extensor carpi radialis longus, brevis, and extensor communis musculature. These are the predominant distal muscle groups active during this phase.

The follow-through phase begins with ball contact and ends with completion of the stroke. The follow-through phase of both the forehand and backhand exhibited continued high activity in the ECRB muscle. The backhand also had moderate levels of biceps activity during the follow-through phase, assisting in the controlled deceleration of elbow extension.

A study by Kelley, Lombardo, Pink, Perry, and Giangarra (1994) compared EMG activity of the extensor digitorum communis, extensor carpi radialis longus and brevis, pronator teres, and flexor carpi radialis in the dominant elbow of 22 competitive tennis players, eight of whom had lateral epicondylitis (tennis elbow), during execution of a backhand groundstroke. Analysis of the players with lateral epicondylitis identified significantly greater activity in the extensor carpi radialis longus and brevis, pronator teres, and flexor carpi radialis compared to the muscular activity of the backhand groundstroke of competitive players without upper extremity injury. This difference in muscular activity was most pronounced during ball contact and the follow-through phase of the backhand groundstroke. Faulty mechanical execution of the backhand corresponded to the increased muscular activity patterns in the injured players. The characteristic "leading-elbow" backhand and open racquet face at impact were additionally identified among the injured players using video analysis.

TABLE 1.4 Muscular Activity Patterns of the Distal Upper Extremity During Tennis Groundstrokes: Mean Percentage of MMT of the Forehand (FH) and Backhand (BH) Groundstrokes

Stage	ECRL FH	BH	ECRB FH	BH	Pronator teres FH	BH	Brachialis FH	BH	Biceps FH	BH	EDC FH	BH	FCR FH	BH
Preparation	26	6	24	7	12	4	14	8	21	13	17	16	15	5
Acceleration	48	48	58	60	24	33	55	31	55	35	44	69	36	19
Follow-through early:	15	39	49	47	22	28	16	36	48	16	31	33	34	26
late:	29*	10	27	16	7	7	9	12	17	5	22	17	5	7

*Follow-through is broken down into two phases in these two motions. ECRB = Extensor carpi radialis brevis, ECRL = Extensor carpi radialis longus, EDC = Extensor digitorum communis, FCR = Flexor carpi radialis.

Use of a two-handed backhand has been advocated for players with upper extremity injury, particularly tennis elbow, because of bilateral upper extremity force generation and load sharing (Nirschl & Sobel, 1981). A recent study by Giangarra, Conroy, Jobe, Pink, and Perry(1993) compared the muscular activity of the elbow, forearm, and wrist during one- and two-handed backhands. Significantly greater flexor carpi radialis muscular activity was measured in the dominant arm during preparation and greater pronator teres activation during acceleration. No significant difference was noted in wrist extensor activity between the one- and two-handed backhand. The greater pronator teres activity in the dominant arm may be the result of the greater degree of forearm pronation in the two-handed stroke, and the presence of the nondominant arm during acceleration may necessitate a countering pronatory muscle activation to stabilize the racquet. As no significant difference was found in extensor activity, the authors postulate that the primary advantage of the two-handed stroke may lie in increased control and range-of-motion limitation of the upper extremity distal segments afforded by addition of the second arm. The additional extremity provided a checkrein of sorts against inappropriate elbow, forearm, and wrist movement patterns.

Golf Swing

The golf swing is typically broken down into the following phases: takeaway, forward swing, acceleration, and follow-through (Jobe, Moynes, & Antonelli, 1986). Takeaway begins with the initiation of motion from the address position and continues to the end of the backswing. Wrist flexor activity is minimal during this phase, with extensor activity averaging 33.6 percent of maximum voluntary contraction (MVC) (Glazebrook, Curwin, Islam, Kozey, & Stanish, 1994). The forward swing phase extends from the end of backswing until the club becomes horizontal, with the acceleration phase lasting from the horizontal club position to ball contact. Muscular activity averages 35 to 45 percent of MVC in the wrist flexors and extensors, respectively (Glazebrook et al., 1994). Ball contact is characterized by relatively high levels of wrist flexor activity (91 percent of MVC), which is commonly referred to as the flexor burst (Glazebrook et al., 1994). The wrist extensors are also more active during ball contact, with a mean level of 58.8 percent. The follow-through phase begins at ball contact and terminates at the end of the golf swing. Wrist extension activity levels are nearly identical during the acceleration and follow-through phases, with wrist flexor activity decreasing to between 60 and 70 percent of MVC following the flexor burst (Glazebrook et al., 1994).

Glazebrook et al. (1994) studied the muscular activity patterns of normal golfers and those with medial epicondylitis. Using surface electrodes applied to the common flexor and extensor tendons at the elbow, significantly greater wrist flexor muscle activity was reported in the golfers with medial epicondylitis during the takeaway and forward swing/acceleration phases. No significant difference was noted in muscular activity during ball contact or follow-through, or with the wrist extensor musculature.

This increase in muscular activity from the injured or overloaded muscle tendon unit is consistent with findings reported with the backhand groundstroke in subjects with lateral epicondylitis. Interestingly, the increased wrist flexor activity measured in subjects with medial epicondylitis is found during phases that normally are not high in wrist flexor demand or activity levels among asymptomatic golfers. The findings of increased and longer duration muscular activation appear consistently throughout the biomechanical analysis of both injured and novice- to intermediate-level athletes.

Further analysis of muscular activity patterns was performed by Glazebrook et al. (1994) to test the effects of a counterforce brace and larger golf club grip size on wrist flexor muscle activity. The authors found no significant difference with these commonly used intervention strategies among the symptomatic subjects.

Joint Kinematics and Kinetics

Understanding the range of motion of and forces at work on the elbow provides the clinician with a better understanding of injury patterns and stresses involved with rehabilitative exercise. Halls and Travill (1964) implanted transducers in the forearms of cadavers to measure the force distribution of an axial load applied to the elbow. They report that 57 percent of the axial load was transferred to the humerus through the radiocapitellar joint, whereas 43 percent was transmitted through the ulnohumeral joint. Analysis of the forces and joint angular velocities of the elbow during sport-specific movements assists in further understanding the demands placed upon the athletic elbow. Table 1.5 summarizes the angular velocities found in the elbow, forearm, and wrist during various sport-specific activities.

Baseball Pitching

Fleisig and Barrentine (1995) tested healthy professional baseball pitchers using high-speed video digitization. They reported varus torques (acting to resist valgus stresses) at the elbow of 64 newton-meters (N-m) occurring at the time of maximal external rotation of the dominant shoulder. The 64 N-m of torque is higher than those causing failure to the medial collateral ligament in isolated cadaver experiments. Dillman tested 11 cadaver

TABLE 1.5   Joint Angular Velocities of the Elbow, Forearm, and Wrist in Upper Extremity Sport Activities

Movement	Sport activity	Angular velocity	Source
Elbow extension	Baseball pitching	2200°/sec	Feltner & Dapena, 1986
Elbow extension	Baseball pitching	2300°/sec	Werner et al., 1993
Elbow extension	Football pass	1760°/sec	Fleisig & Barrentine, 1995
Elbow extension	Javelin thrust	1900°/sec	Mero et al., 1994
Elbow flexion	Softball pitching	680°/sec	Barrentine, 1994
Elbow extension	Tennis serve	1700°/sec	Dillman, 1991
Elbow extension	Tennis serve	982°/sec	Kibler, 1994
Forearm pronation	Tennis serve	347°/sec	Kibler, 1994
Wrist flexion	Tennis serve	315°/sec	VanGheluwe & Hebbelinck, 1986

elbows to determine the ultimate tensile stress of the ulnar collateral ligament (Fleisig et al., 1989). The ultimate tensile stress was determined to be 642 newtons before failure, which corresponds to 32 N-m of varus torque to resist valgus stress.

The fact that the ulnar collateral ligament alone cannot withstand the focal valgus stresses imparted during throwing confirms the previously discussed concept of dynamic stabilization by the surrounding musculature. Contraction of the triceps and anconeus muscles during the acceleration phase of throwing may reduce stress on the ulnar collateral ligament by compressing the ulnohumeral joint and adding stability (Fleisig & Barrentine, 1995). This reinforces the use of strength and endurance training of the elbow musculature in rehabilitation and preventive conditioning for athletes in these populations.

In comparison, a peak valgus torque (resisting varus stress) of 40 N-m at the elbow occurred just prior to ball release. A compressive force, acting to resist distraction of the elbow, increased slowly throughout the pitching motion from the time of front foot contact until the time of ball release. The maximum value for this compressive force was 780 newtons.

Range of motion of the elbow during throwing is consistently reported from 85° of flexion at the time of maximal external shoulder rotation in the cocking phase to 20° of extension at time of ball release (Werner et al., 1993), and 89° of flexion to 20° of extension is reported by Feltner and Dapena (1986). This elbow range of motion occurs at a rate of 2200° to 2300° per second during acceleration of the throwing motion (Feltner & Dapena, 1986; Werner et al., 1993).

Other Throwing Activities

Throwing a football has been used as an overload activity for baseball pitchers. Although throwing a football and pitching have some similarities, they have measurable differences. During the cocking phase of football throwing, a maximum medial force of 280 newtons and a varus torque of 54 N-m is produced (Fleisig & Barrentine, 1995). A compressive force of 620 newtons is generated during deceleration of the arm.

During arm cocking, a quarterback averages 113° of elbow flexion and extends the elbow at 1760° per second. Compared to a pitcher, a quarterback produces greater medial force to the elbow during cocking, greater anterior force at the shoulder, and less internal rotation and varus torque during arm acceleration. The increased varus torque at the elbow may be related to the greater incidence of medial elbow injuries with baseball pitching compared to throwing a football.

Barrentine (1994) studied the kinetic and kinematic parameters of the elbow during underhand throwing. A compressive force equal to 438 newtons is exerted to resist distraction of the forearm at the elbow. A valgus torque (to resist varus stress at the elbow) is generated that equals 45 N-m to counter the elbow flexion and shoulder internal rotation movement patterns that are used to generate ball velocity when throwing a softball underhand. Although the magnitude of forces at the elbow is smaller with throwing a softball underhand, the repetitive stresses and anatomical differences such as increased carrying angle among female participants may subject the elbow to injury (Fleisig & Barrentine, 1995).

Tennis Serve

Kinematic values similar to those measured with overhand throwing are reported for the tennis serve. Kibler (1994) reports elbow range of motion during the late cocking to acceleration phases to range from 116° of flexion to 20° of extension, with ball impact occurring at a mean of 35° of elbow extension. Forearm pronation/supination ranges from 15° of supination during the cocking phase to 70° of pronation at ball impact. Elbow joint range of motion is much smaller during groundstrokes, with only 11° (46° to 35°) on the forehand and 18° (48° to 30°) on the backhand (Kibler, 1994).

Sprigings, Marshall, Elliott, and Jennings (1994) published a three-dimensional kinematic analysis that clearly demonstrates the important role of the entire upper extremity kinetic chain in the tennis serve. Anatomic rotations of the upper extremity during the serving motion of an elite tennis player were calculated and listed in rank order of contribution to the racquet head velocity achieved. Internal rotation of the shoulder ranked first at 8 meters per second, followed by wrist flexion at 7 meters per second. Shoulder horizontal adduction at 6.5 meters per second and forearm pronation at 4 meters per second were also major contributors. Wrist ulnar deviation and elbow extension were not significant contributors to racquet head velocity.

Cohen, Mont, Campbell, Vogelstein, and Loewy (1994) studied 40 elite-level male tennis players by evaluating the relationship between serving velocity and anthropometric data and extremity strength. Statistically significant relationships were found between serving velocity and increased wrist flexion, shoulder flexion, and internal rotation range of motion on the dominant shoulder. Isokinetically measured elbow extension strength and the external/internal unilateral strength ratio both concentrically and eccentrically were statistically related to serving velocity in this population.

The summation and integration of each individual segment of the throwing and serving motion is of vital overall importance. The scientific evidence presented in these key studies provides rationale for the use of total arm strength rehabilitation for athletic elbow injuries.

Weightlifting and Other Exercise Movements

Donkers, An, Chao, and Morrey (1993) studied the forces acting on the elbow during a push-up exercise. The peak compressive force is equal to 45 percent of body weight with the hands in the normal push-up position. The elbow compressive forces were decreased by placing the hands farther apart or in a more superior position. A one-arm push-up exercise increased compressive force 31 percent more than the two-arm push-up. Valgus torque increases 54 percent with the hands in a superior position or 42 percent when one arm is used during the push-up.

Weightlifting produces stresses on the elbow that are range-of-motion dependent (Donkers et al., 1993; Werner & An, 1994). With the elbow in an extended position, the force is directed anteriorly, whereas a flexed elbow position produces posteriorly directed stresses. The greatest magnitude for resultant force, which can be more than three times body weight, occurs at approximately 30° of elbow flexion.

CHAPTER | 2

Etiology of Overuse Elbow Injuries and Anatomical Adaptations in Athletes

Evaluation and treatment of the injured athletic elbow require a thorough understanding of the etiological factors of elbow overuse injuries. Research identifying the characteristic anatomical adaptations in athletes with unilaterally dominant upper extremity use serves to educate the clinician on the differences between normal and abnormal findings in this population.

Humeral Epicondylitis (Tennis Elbow)

Humeral epicondylitis, which has been cited in the literature as early as 1873 by Runge, is a common overuse injury known today as tennis elbow. In 1936, Cyriax listed 26 possible causes of tennis elbow (Cyriax & Cyriax, 1983). Debate among medical professionals continues regarding its etiology (Nirschl, 1993). Differential diagnoses include ulnar nerve neuropraxia, carpal tunnel syndrome, radial nerve entrapment, osteochondritis dissecans, joint calcification, osteoarthritis, periostitis, orbital ligament abnormalities, and synovial fringe impingement (Bernhang, Dehner, & Fogarty, 1974; Nirschl, 1984). Gross and microscopic examination of the pathological tissue has led to a better clinical understanding of tennis elbow.

23

In a normal tendon under microscopic examination, longitudinally arrayed fascicles of dense collagen fibers with slender, elongated fibroblastic cells known as tenocytes should be found (Kiriti & Unthoff, 1980). In the common extensor tendon with tennis elbow, microscopic analysis shows irregularly distributed mesenchymal cells and disarrayed and fragmented fascicles, along with newly formed vascular channels. These microscopic signs found in injured tendons suggest an intrinsic healing mechanism in the tendon itself.

Goldie's analysis noted hypervascularization of the extensor aponeurosis and an increased quantity of free nerve endings in the subtendinous space (Goldie, 1964). Nirschl (1977) states that the characteristic pathology is a granulation response with fibroblastic and vascular proliferation associated with general edema and calcification in later stages. Gross examination of the extensor carpi radialis brevis (ECRB) tendon reveals grayish, immature scar tissue appearing shiny, edematous, and friable. Nirschl has termed this characteristic invasion "angiofibroblastic hyperplasia."

Leadbetter (1992) describes sports-induced overuse tendon injury in the wrist extensor, Achilles, patellar, and rotator cuff tendons as occurring from repetitive eccentric loads on muscle tendon units that cross more than one joint and have a tenuous blood supply. Figure 2.1 outlines Leadbetter's (1992) theoretical pathway of sports-induced inflammatory response. This response is a time-dependent process characterized by vascular, chemical, and cellular events within the tendon leading to tissue repair, regeneration, or scar formation. The repair of soft tissue or tendon injury has been defined as the replacement of damaged cells and extracellular matrices with new cells and matrices.

A tendon's response to injury represents a failure of the cellular matrix adaptation to overload. The microscopic tendon injury is perceived as immunologically subclinical by the immune system and is not of significant magnitude and character to stimulate the structured, interacting sequence of an inflammatory response (Whiteside & Andrews, 1995). Instead, there is a proliferation of tendon intrasubstance and degenerative changes in the tendon, including cellular atrophy, decreased number of active cells, and decreased protein synthesis.

The cumulative cell matrix adaptive response injuries to tendons described by Leadbetter (1992) consist of acute (sudden onset) and chronic (slow, insidious onset, often with a subclinical spectrum of structural damage leading to injury) and are outlined in figure 2.2. This description of tendon injury has prompted the term "tendinosis," defined as a focal region of intratendinous degeneration. A prominent source of degeneration is cell atrophy, which is caused by disuse, immobilization, and age, resulting in a decrease in size and function. This degenerative process responsible for tendon injury is treatable and responds to passive mobilization and controlled use of load. Slowing the degenerative process and facilitat-

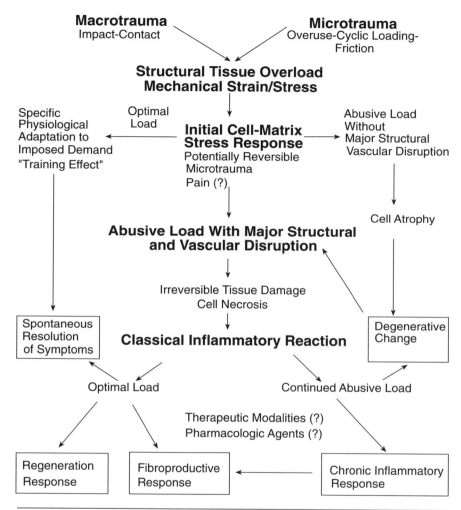

FIGURE 2.1 Schema of the theoretical pathways of sports-induced inflammatory response. Reprinted from Leadbetter et al. 1990.

ing the reparative mechanisms are primary goals in the nonoperative treatment of overuse tendon injury in the elbow.

A thorough review of the literature identifies humeral epicondylitis as an extra-articular, tendinous overuse injury resulting from both degenerative and inflammatory processes (Leadbetter, 1992; Nirschl, 1977, 1984). Repetitive stresses imparted to the upper extremity of the athlete can eventually result in excessive vascular granulation and an impaired healing environment within the injured tendon. Nociceptive and mechanoreceptor stimulation result in the characteristic pain responses that limit

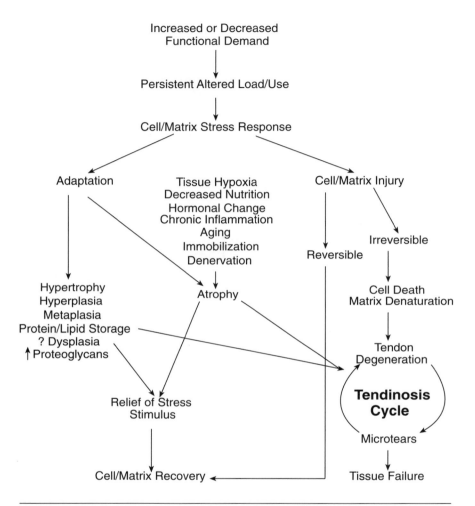

FIGURE 2.2   Cell matrix response to change in functional level. In this model, tendinosis results from a failed cell matrix adaptation to excessive changes in load use. Such failure is modified by both intrinsic and extrinsic factors. Reprinted from Leadbetter 1992.

performance of both ADL and sport activity. Humeral epicondylitis is normally classified by its location on the humerus, lateral or medial.

Lateral Epicondylitis

In 1964, Goldie published a comprehensive analysis of tennis elbow describing lateral epicondylitis as inflammation of the extensor carpi radialis brevis and extensor communis aponeurosis at the lateral epicondyle as well as its subtendinous triangular space at the lateral condyle.

The primary structure involved with lateral epicondylitis is the muscle tendon unit of the extensor carpi radialis brevis. The extensor carpi radialis longus, extensor communis, and extensor carpi ulnaris can also be involved (Nirschl & Sobel, 1981). It is clinically important to note that the ECRB originates on the lateral inferior aspect of the lateral epicondyle and is the most lateral of the extensor group (figure 2.3). It is covered by the extensor carpi radialis longus, which originates from the lateral supracondylar column just below the origin of the brachioradialis and above the ECRB (Morrey, 1993). The ECRB is exclusively a wrist extensor and has no effect on radial or ulnar deviation. The extensor communis originates from the common tendon just ulnar or medial to the ECRB. The extensor carpi ulnaris has two heads of origin. The humeral origin from the lateral epicondyle is

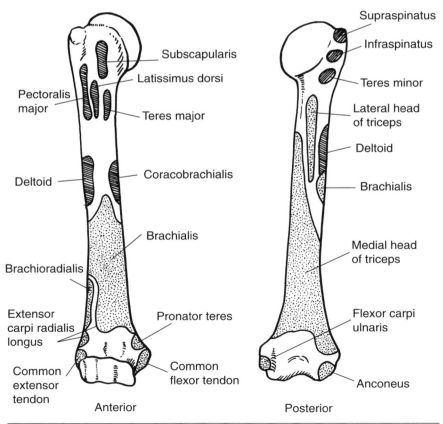

FIGURE 2.3   Humeral origin and insertion of muscles affecting the elbow joint.

the most medial on the common extensor tendon, and the ulnar attachment is along the aponeurosis of the anconeus muscle.

Force overloads to the extensor musculature due to intrinsic muscular contraction, as well as extrinsic factors such as a stretch-induced trauma from sport-specific performance patterns, are reported to stress these structures progressively. A mechanical disadvantage to stress overload exists due to the inherent structure of the medially sloping lateral condyle, which creates a fulcrum effect of the prominent radial head. This leverage effect, coupled with the increased tension of the lateral musculature with the arm in the pronated position during the backhand groundstroke and other sport-specific and ADL activities, makes the lateral elbow susceptible to overload stresses. The repetitive nature of these stresses and the failure of the dynamic muscular supporting structure to function effectively in an endurance-oriented fashion create a continuum of disability.

Medial Epicondylitis

Medial epicondylitis most commonly involves the pronator teres, flexor carpi radialis, and flexor carpi ulnaris, all of which originate from a common site on the medial epicondyle (figure 2.3). The pronator teres has two heads of origin. The larger humeral origin is the most proximal on the anterosuperior aspect of the medial epicondyle. The ulnar origin of the pronator teres is on the coronoid. The median nerve passes between these two heads of origin. The flexor carpi radialis originates just distal to the pronator teres on the common flexor tendon, on the anteroinferior aspect of the medial epicondyle. The flexor carpi ulnaris is the most posterior of the tendons originating on the medial epicondyle and has a second, larger head of origin from the medial border of the coronoid. The ulnar nerve enters and innervates the muscle between these two heads of origin, giving off two or three motor branches.

Posterior Tennis Elbow

A third form of tennis elbow is described in the literature but is not technically humeral epicondylitis. Posterior tennis elbow involves the triceps tendon as it inserts into the olecranon of the ulna (Nirschl & Sobel, 1981). It is caused by repetitive stress to the triceps tendon, most notably during the acceleration phase of throwing and the tennis serve. Inappropriate mechanics on the backhand groundstroke, specifically using a whipping-type extension movement at the elbow, can also cause this form of tennis elbow.

Distribution of Humeral Epicondylitis

According to Nirschl and Sobel (1981), distribution of epicondylitis occurrence is dependent on skill level, with recreational and novice players suffering a 90 percent lateral and 10 percent medial distribution. Inappropriate mechanics on the backhand groundstroke, specifically the leading-elbow backhand, is cited as one of the most likely causes of lateral epicondylitis in tennis. In highly skilled players, the distribution is reversed to 75 percent medial and 25 percent lateral. This increase in medial epicondylitis in skilled players is most often attributed to the stresses imparted to the medial aspect of the elbow during powerful and repetitive serving.

Specific patterns of humeral epicondylitis are reported in golfers (Nirschl & Sobel, 1981). Medial epicondylitis, often termed "golfer's elbow," is most commonly found in the right elbow of a right-handed golfer. The forearm pronator and wrist flexor muscle activity during acceleration of the golf swing can load these tendons repetitively. Consequently, lateral epicondylitis is commonly associated with the left elbow in the right-handed golfer. A further discussion of specific mechanisms of injury will be presented in discussions on interval sport return programs and evaluation of pathomechanics later in this text.

Ulnar Collateral Ligament Injury

The kinetic and kinematic descriptions of the elbow during throwing (see chapter 1) clearly demonstrate the excessive valgus stresses imparted to the medial elbow during late cocking and acceleration and highlight the primary responsibility of and load on the anterior aspect of the medial collateral ligament. Injury to the ulnar or medial collateral ligament most commonly occurs in the throwing elbow, whether from baseball pitching, javelin throwing, or the tennis serve. Poor mechanics, lack of flexibility and overall conditioning, as well as fatigue from overuse can all have a cumulative effect that leads to a decrease in active muscular protection of the medial elbow and hence greater stress to the ulnar collateral ligament (Jobe & Kvitne, 1991).

Progressive damage to the ulnar collateral ligament initially appears as edema and inflammation within the ligament. Consistent with ligament sprains in other anatomical locations throughout the body, pain, localized tenderness, and swelling about the medial elbow are present. With continued stress to the ligament, dissociation of the ligament fibers occurs, progressing to calcification and ossification. The scar tissue and ossification within the ligament increase stress and, over time, can lead to attenuation and subsequent rupture of the ligament. The ligament can be avulsed from the ulnar insertion or, less likely, tear midsubstance. The ligament is less likely to be avulsed from the medial epicondyle.

Attenuation of the ligament can lead to joint instability, which compromises performance and can subject the elbow to further injury. These injuries are discussed in the following sections.

Ulnar Nerve Injury (Neuritis)

Injury to the ulnar nerve is best described by the anatomical pathway it descends. The winding course of the ulnar nerve begins 8 cm proximal to the medial epicondyle as the nerve travels from the anterior to posterior compartment of the brachium, penetrating a thick fibrous raphe termed the arcade of Struthers. This arcade is formed by the medial head of the triceps, medial intermuscular septum, and deep fascia of the arm (Jobe, Fanton, & Ellatrache, 1993). The arcade of Struthers can cause entrapment primarily or from tethering after transposition of the nerve postoperatively.

The ulnar nerve continues distally and winds behind the medial epicondyle, entering the cubital groove. The groove is formed by the ulnar collateral ligament, the medial edge of the trochlea, the medial epicondyle, and the roof, which is formed by the cubital tunnel retinaculum (see figure 1.6). The cubital tunnel retinaculum also acts as a source of origin for the flexor carpi ulnaris muscle, which the nerve passes through as it continues distally. For every 45° of elbow flexion, the cubital tunnel retinaculum must stretch 5 mm, and at 90° of flexion, the proximal edge of the retinaculum becomes taut. This action, coupled with a relaxation and subsequent bulging of the ulnar collateral ligament, produces a reduction in the volume of the cubital tunnel.

Additional tension in the ulnar nerve is produced with elbow flexion (4.7 mm elongation) and with triceps contraction (7 mm medially). The ulnar nerve is not a static structure, and with repetitive movements of the elbow, friction and sliding of the nerve in this anatomic location can cause local perineural damage (Apfelberg & Larson, 1973). Inflammation of the ulnar nerve, termed neuritis, can occur from the mechanical stresses of repetitive upper extremity use, especially in the presence of anatomical compromise such as muscular inflexibility, bony encroachment, and ligamentous instability.

Attenuation of the ulnar collateral ligament can place additional stress on the ulnar nerve, resulting in elbow instability due to valgus stress. Increased tension on the ulnar nerve can also occur during throwing due to the elevation of intraneural pressure from the combined movements of shoulder abduction, 90° of elbow flexion, and extension of the wrist. Pressures of up to six times that in the relaxed nerve could result from the combined upper extremity movement patterns during throwing or the tennis serve (Pechan & Julius, 1975).

Congenital absence of the cubital tunnel retinaculum can cause dislocation of the ulnar nerve from the cubital groove. Friction neuritis can result from the hypermobility of the nerve as it partially or completely dislocates around the medial epicondyle.

The ulnar nerve's course is further described in the discussion of ulnar nerve injury in chapter 6. Ulnar nerve zones at the medial epicondyle are broken down into zone 1 (proximal to the medial epicondyle), zone 2 (at the medial epicondyle), and zone 3 (distal to the medial epicondyle). Symptoms of ulnar nerve neuropraxia have been reported by Nirschl in 60 percent of surgical candidates for medial epicondylitis. The most common site of involvement has been in zone 3 near the penetration of the nerve through the flexor carpi ulnaris arcade. Symptoms are mainly sensory and include the ring and fifth finger, without distortion of motor function.

Osteochondral Injuries (Osteophytes/Loose Bodies)

Osseous injuries in the athletic elbow are generally classified into medial tension, lateral compression, and valgus extension overload. Within these three classifications are acute fracture and chronic manifestations of overuse injury.

Medial Tension

In response to valgus stress, the medial aspect of the elbow can develop traction spurs or osteophytes of the medial epicondyle and coronoid (Bennett, 1959; Indelicato et al., 1979; Slocum, 1978). Figure 2.4 portrays the valgus overload stress to the medial elbow and the location of potential medial tensile injury. Injury to the ulnar collateral ligament, ulnar nerve, and flexor-pronator muscle tendon unit are considered medial tension or tensile overload injuries according to this classification.

Lateral Compression

Osteochondritis dissecans of the radiocapitellar joint can be present due to the focal lateral compressive stresses associated with throwing, especially in the adolescent aged 10 to 15 years. One theory is that compressive forces

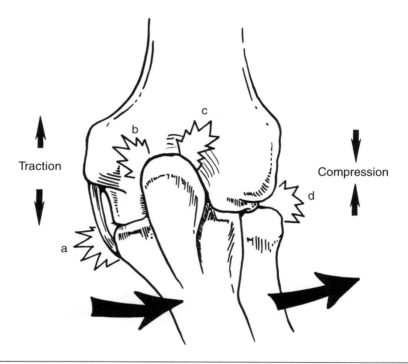

FIGURE 2.4 Anatomical diagram of the effects of valgus stress on the elbow. Arrows represent the valgus stress and rotation that occurs during the acceleration phase of throwing or the tennis serve: (a) medial aspect (traction), (b) contact of the posteromedial aspect of the olecranon leading to osteochondral injury, (c) loose body formation, and (d) lateral aspect (compression). Adapted from Indelicato et al. 1979.

cause arterial injury and subsequent bone death. Hypertrophy of both the capitellum and radial head, as well as loose body formation, are also described as lateral compression injuries (Joyce et al., 1995).

Compression of the lateral aspect of the elbow is especially common with attenuation of the medial collateral ligament in the throwing arm, where increased load transmission occurs across the radiocapitellar joint, leading to chondromalacia of the articular surfaces and ultimately progressing to more severe degeneration and osteochondritis dissecans (Joyce et al., 1995).

Valgus Extension Overload

Valgus stress with medial elbow instability, combined with repetitive extension overload, can result in posteromedial olecranon osteophyte formation due to impingement of the posteromedial aspect of the proximal ulna against the trochlea and olecranon fossa of the distal humerus. One finding often preceding osteophyte formation on the olecranon is development of chondromalacia on the medial aspect of the trochlear groove on the humerus (Joyce et al., 1995). Erosion to subchondral bone is often seen when olecranon osteophytes are just beginning.

The development of posterior loose bodies and fibrous scar tissue deposition is also reported in the posterior aspect of the elbow (Wilson, Andrews, Blackburn, & McCluskey, 1983). Most loose bodies are broken spurs that formed initially in the impingement of the posterior aspect of the olecranon and trochlea or osteocartilaginous fragments from an osteochondritis lesion of the capitellum (Joyce et al., 1995). The incidence of loose bodies in the elbow in the normal population is unknown; however, 39 percent of professional baseball players have been reported to have loose bodies at the time of elbow surgery (Joyce et al., 1995).

Growth Plate Injury

Repetitive valgus extension stresses applied to the immature athlete can lead to injury of the epiphyseal growth plates (physes). Acute injury to the medial epicondylar apophysis can be in the form of an avulsion, with chronic stress leading to traction apophysitis. Epiphyseal separation will occur in adolescents instead of rupture of the ulnar collateral ligament (Joyce et al., 1995). The cartilaginous growth plate represents the weak link, and before fusion of the secondary ossification center, strong forceful contraction of the flexor/pronator musculature can cause epiphyseal separation.

Acute avulsion and chronic apophysitis of the olecranon apophysis from forceful contraction and stress produced by the triceps has also been described in the literature (Morrey, 1993). Additional growth-related injuries in the adolescent are reported, but injuries to the medial epicondylar and olecranon physes are most commonly associated with sports-related activities.

The growth plate is a cartilaginous disk between the epiphysis and metaphysis of the bone. The site of separation of the growth plate is frequently between calcified and uncalcified cartilage matrix. The relatively small amount of calcified matrix at this level accounts for the relative weakness of the growth plate, making the area vulnerable to injury with repeated stress. The Salter-Harris classification of growth plate injuries is the generally accepted classification system. Founded on the pathology of injury, this system is well suited to the accurate verbal description of an injury and provides an excellent guide to rational treatment (Rang, 1983).

In a type I Salter-Harris fracture, the epiphysis separates completely from the metaphysis. The germinal cell layer remains with the epiphysis and the calcified layer remains with the metaphysis. If the periosteum is not torn, there is no displacement. Type I injuries usually occur from shearing, torsion, or avulsion forces. An apophysis, which is a prominent process projecting from the surface of a bone that it has never been separated from or movable upon (Rang, 1983), is usually avulsed.

In a type II Salter-Harris injury, the plane of cleavage passes through much of the growth plate before the fracture travels through the metaphysis. The fracture is produced from a lateral displacement force that tears the periosteum on one side and leaves it intact in the region of the metaphyseal fragment. Type III injuries are seen in partially closed growth plates, with the plane of separation along the growth plate before entering the joint through a fracture of the epiphysis. The fracture itself is intra-articular and requires accurate reduction to prevent malarticulation. The type IV injury fracture line passes from the joint surface, across the epiphysis, and into the metaphysis. The most common example is a fracture of the lateral condyle of the humerus (Rang, 1983). Finally, in a type V injury, the growth plate is crushed, extinguishing further growth, with all or most of the growth plate being affected (Salter & Harris, 1963).

Ossification Centers of the Throwing Elbow

Ossification centers of primary importance to the athletic throwing elbow are the medial epicondyle and olecranon ossification centers. The medial epicondylar ossification center is the second ossification center to appear at age 4. It develops slowly and is the last center to unite with the humeral shaft, as late as 15 to 16 years of age (Graviss & Hoffman, 1993). Due to the large valgus stresses and high-intensity muscular forces from the tendinous attachment of the flexor-pronator muscle group, the young throwing or racquet sports athlete can develop problems at the medial epicondyle.

The olecranon ossification center usually develops at approximately 9 years of age and begins to unite at age 14. The high-intensity muscular contraction of the triceps through its insertion on the olecranon during the acceleration phase of the throwing and serving motions may create problems in this region. These osseous injuries further support standard radiographic evaluation of the elbow during the comprehensive evaluation process prior to commencement of a rehabilitation program.

Anatomical Adaptations of the Elbow in Unilaterally Dominant Athletes

Anatomical adaptations are characteristic findings reported in the research literature that differ from accepted normal anatomical structure or relationships found in the normal population. Anatomical adaptations are thought to provide insight into both the location and magnitude of stresses to an athlete's body, as well as the body's reaction or adaptation to these stresses. Knowledge of sport-specific anatomical adaptations of the elbow assists the clinician in both evaluation and treatment of the injured athlete.

Range-of-Motion Adaptations

King, Brelsford, and Tullos (1969) initially reported that the dominant elbow in 50 percent of professional baseball pitchers had a flexion contracture, and 30 percent had a cubitus valgus angular deformity. They believed that this flexion contracture prevented olecranon impingement during the follow-through phase of throwing. Slocum (1978) postulates that the elbow flexion contracture commonly seen is due to interstitial muscle fibrosis in the flexor-pronator group caused by chronic microtears from throwing. Indelicato et al. (1979) suggest that another etiology for the flexion contracture lies in the inflammatory response of the anterior capsule of the elbow, leading to a secondary contracture from repetitive forceful extension.

Chinn, Priest, and Kent (1974) measured 53 internationally ranked tennis players and found significant elbow flexion contractures in males but no cubitus valgus deformity. Ellenbecker (1992b) also found statistically significant flexion contractures in the dominant elbow of elite male junior tennis players and in competitive senior male (mean 6°) tennis players (Ellenbecker & Roetert, 1994). A consistent loss of dominant-arm elbow and wrist extension range of motion was also goniometrically measured in elite junior tennis players (Ellenbecker, 1992a).

Osseous Adaptations

Priest, Jones, & Nagel (1974) studied 84 top-ranked tennis professionals. Through x-ray evaluation of the players' dominant and nondominant elbows, the researchers found soft tissue ossification, alterations of muscle and ligament attachments, and hypertrophic bone growth. In male players, an average of 6.5 changes in the dominant arm were found. Males had twice as many medial elbow region changes as lateral, with the coronoid process of the ulna being the primary site of hypertrophy or spurring. They also reported posterior and lateral trochlear osteophyte formation from the valgus extension overload of the service motion. An average cortical increase of 44 percent was found in the anterior aspect of the humeral cortex in the dominant arm, with an increase of 11 percent in the radius and ulna.

Huddleston, Rockwell, Kulund, and Harrison (1980) measured the bone mass in the dominant arm of 35 active senior tennis players aged 70 to 84 and found increased bone mineralization in the radius. In a more recent study, Krahl, Michaelis, Pieper, Quack, and Montag (1994) studied the dominant and nondominant arms of 20 high-ranking professional tennis players between the ages of 13 and 26. Radiographic examinations of the players showed significantly greater bone density in the dominant arm as well as an increase in bone diameter and length of the ulna and second metacarpal. The authors attribute this unilateral response to the biopositive adaptive reaction from the mechanical stimulation of the tennis-playing extremity as well as the associated hyperemia from tennis play.

Additional research on unilateral bone mass development in female national-level tennis and squash players demonstrates the effects of unilateral exercise. Kannus (1995) studied 105 Finnish national-level tennis and squash players and compared them to 50 controls. Significantly greater bone mineral content was found in the dominant humerus and radius among the tennis and squash players. Greater dominant arm strength and circumference were also found in the racquet sport players, with no significant difference in control subjects.

One additional unique finding in this study was the two to four times greater dominant/nondominant difference in bone mineral content among racquet sport athletes who started their playing careers before or at menarche compared to those athletes whose playing careers started after menarche. This study not only provides evidence supporting physical activity, but indicates that physical activity during prepubescent years is crucial for maximizing bone mass.

Anthropometrics

Chinn et al. (1974) found significantly greater dominant forearm girths in elite male tennis players, with similar anthropometric findings reported by Kulund, Rockwell, and Brubaker (1979) in senior competitive players and by Carlson and Cera (1984) in the forearm and biceps of elite junior male and female players. Consistent with dominant arm muscular hypertrophy is the reported finding of greater grip strength on the dominant (racquet) arm when compared to the nondominant (Carlson & Cera, 1984; Chinn et al., 1974; Ellenbecker, 1991; Kulund et al., 1979; Vodak, Savin, & Haskell, 1980).

CHAPTER | 3 |

Diagnostic Tests for the Elbow

In addition to a thorough clinical exam, the complete evaluation of the athlete with an injured elbow normally includes numerous diagnostic tests. A general understanding of the types of diagnostic tests typically applied, as well as the rationale for selecting the appropriate tests, will benefit the rehabilitation specialist.

Radiographs

Initial evaluation of an athlete's elbow should include basic screening radiographs. The basic views recommended are an anteroposterior view in full extension and a lateral view at 90° of flexion. Other helpful views include an axial view and the oblique views, both left and right. Plain, or unenhanced, radiographs are used in the proper evaluation of traumatic injuries and to diagnose chronic abnormalities of the elbow. They are essential in ruling out fractures and dislocations. Radiographs also reveal degenerative changes such as osteophytes and other abnormalities such as ossific loose bodies and calcific tendinitis.

Plain radiographs play an essential role in identifying osseous abnormalities that often cannot be delineated with even the most thorough clinical examination by a therapist or trainer. They also assist in ruling out serious osseous injury as well as disease processes such as tumors. One example of how the plain radiograph can influence the rehabilitation of an overuse injury is with humeral epicondylitis. Frequently, a plain radiograph shows a bone spur on the epicondyle in a mature tennis player. The presence of this spur can help explain why it is taking a long time for the patient's pain and discomfort to diminish. The patient with humeral epicondylitis is

normally an excellent candidate for rehabilitation, but when a spur is identified on a radiograph, the patient's prognosis can be calculated more real-
istically.

Comparison radiographic views of the opposite elbow can be helpful in
diagnosing elbow injuries in the younger athlete. This comparison is especially beneficial when comparing abnormalities of the physeal (growth)
plates.

Stress Radiographs

Although pain and proper positioning can make stress radiographs difficult to obtain, stress views can be very helpful in diagnosing instability
and physeal injuries about the elbow. A recent study by Goitz, Rijke,
Andrews, Phillips, and McCue (1994) has shown graded stress radiography using a modified Telos GA-II/E stress device (Austin & Associates,
Fallston, MD) to be a useful, noninvasive method of evaluating medial
elbow pain in the throwing athlete and, in particular, for testing the status
of the medial ulnar collateral ligament (figure 3.1).

Stress radiographs are performed with the elbow in 25° of flexion to
unlock the olecranon from the surrounding bony fossa. Full supination of

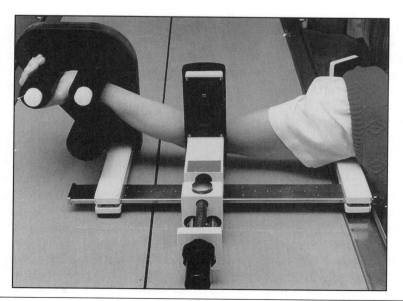

FIGURE 3.1   Position and technique for performing stress radiography for the elbow.
A valgus stress is applied to the left elbow with a Telos stress device.

the forearm is also used to ensure a reproducible testing position that closely approximates the position used during the clinical stress test of the medial ulnar collateral ligament. Stress radiographs are essential to a thorough evaluation of the throwing athlete with acute or chronic medial elbow pain. The cost-effectiveness and noninvasive nature of this test make it attractive to the examiner and injured athlete alike.

Contrast Arthrography

Contrast dye arthrography has long been used to help diagnose elbow injuries. Leakage of dye from within or through the capsule may indicate injury to the ligamentous structures. This test has also helped detect intra-articular loose bodies by further delineating the capsular boundaries of the joint. Unfortunately, contrast arthrography is invasive and can have some associated discomfort. Some individuals may also be allergic to certain dye substances. A thorough medical history for prior allergic reactions should therefore be obtained before testing.

Contrast arthrography is performed by inserting a needle into the joint capsule, most commonly the lateral side of the joint in a location termed the soft spot. Following injection, the extremity is extended and flexed and taken through the available ranges of motion to mobilize the injected dye within the joint capsule. Radiographic procedures are then performed, including plain radiographs, computed tomography (CT) scans, and magnetic resonance imaging (MRI). The dye serves to enhance the image on the previously mentioned studies.

Computed Tomography

Computed tomography has been used in conjunction with contrast arthrography to delineate elbow pathologic conditions. It has been useful in evaluating osteochondritis dissecans, stress fractures, loose bodies (intra- and extra-articular), bony and chondral defects, and medial ulnar collateral ligament injuries. The CT-arthrogram combination can uncover a defect in the inner layer (undersurface) of the MCL with the intact external layer, seen during arthroscopic evaluation (Timmerman & Andrews, 1994c).

In a prospective study of 25 baseball pitchers, Timmerman, Schwartz, and Andrews (1994) used both computed tomography and magnetic resonance imaging to evaluate the elbow prior to surgery. CT arthrogram detected abnormalities in 12 of the 14 patients with ulnar collateral ligament injury (86 percent sensitivity), whereas MRI revealed abnormalities in 8 of 14 patients (57 percent sensitivity). In another study, Timmerman et al. (1994) described a "T-sign" visible with CT arthrogram. The "T-sign" represents an undersurface tear of the ulnar collateral ligament, with dye leaking around the detachment of the ulnar collateral ligament from its bony insertion but contained within the intact superficial layer of the ulnar collateral ligament and joint capsule.

Although both computed tomography and MRI are reliable diagnostic tools for evaluation of the athlete with a complete tear of the ulnar collateral ligament, a CT arthrogram is the test of choice for detecting partial undersurface tears of the ulnar collateral ligament.

Magnetic Resonance Imaging (MRI)

Soft tissue structures are usually delineated well enough by MRI that the integrity of capsular and ligamentous structures about the elbow can be evaluated. MRI can reveal damage or potency of muscles and tendons such as distal biceps tendon ruptures. Vascular changes in the bony structures about the elbow can be evaluated with MRI as well. In particular, any osteochondrosis or osteochondritis dissecans of the radiocapitellar joint can be evaluated. MRI imaging was used in a study of medial elbow injuries in 11 baseball pitchers; four patients ultimately underwent surgery where MRI-suspected tears of the medial ulnar collateral ligament were confirmed (Andrews & Soffer, 1994; Timmerman, Schwartz, & Andrews, 1994).

Although arthrogram-enhanced MRI can be used in the elbow, we believe stress radiographs to be more reliable and cost-effective in the evaluation of medial instability of the elbow.

Differential Diagnosis

To ensure an accurate diagnosis of the injured elbow, conditions other than those most commonly seen from overuse in the athletic elbow must be excluded. Table 3.1 lists diagnoses that must be considered and ruled out prior to final diagnosis of an overuse injury in the athletic elbow.

A common differential diagnosis discussed in the literature for lateral elbow pain is posterior interosseous nerve entrapment, also known as radial tunnel syndrome (Roles & Mawdsley, 1972). Distal to the lateral epicondyle of the humerus, the extensor carpi radialis brevis forms an immediate anterolateral relationship with the posterior interosseous nerve and can groove the nerve during forearm pronation. Fascial sheaths present in this location can also tighten around the nerve. Immediately distal to this

TABLE 3.1   Differential Diagnoses for the Elbow

Medial elbow pain	Lateral elbow pain
Medial epicondyle avulsion	Lateral epicondyle avulsion
Anterior interosseous nerve entrapment	Radial nerve entrapment
Ulnar nerve entrapment	Radial head fracture
T1 radiculopathy	C6 radiculopathy
	Rheumatoid arthritis

origin of the extensor carpi radialis brevis, the posterior interosseous nerve passes beneath the fibrous edge of the superficial oblique portion of the supinator muscle. The nerve enters the muscle, dividing it into its two portions. This fibrous region, termed the arcade of Frohse by Frohse and Frankel in 1908, is repeatedly reported as a site of compression or entrapment of the posterior interosseous nerve during passive pronation of the forearm. Additional locations of entrapment for the posterior interosseous nerve are the leash of Henry, the radial recurrent vessels anterior to the lateral epicondyle, and a fibrous band at the distal edge of the supinator muscle (Morrey, 1993).

Clinical signs of posterior interosseous nerve entrapment include reproduction of pain with resisted supination of the injured extremity and with passive pronation range of motion, as well as a region of tenderness just distal to the lateral epicondyle itself (Wadsworth, 1987). Weakness and pain with resisted supination rather than wrist extension are characteristic clinical findings in the patient with posterior interosseous nerve entrapment syndrome (Galloway, DeMaio, & Mangine, 1992). Kamien (1990) adds to the list of common clinical findings weakness of finger extension at the metacarpophalangeal joints of the radial three fingers with a patch of sensory loss over the first web space between the thumb and index finger.

Roles and Mawdsley's (1972) main evidence for entrapment of the posterior interosseous nerve as a cause of lateral elbow pain has been the relief following surgical release and decompression of the radial tunnel. Other sources, however, suggest that nerve entrapment may not be that likely a cause of lateral elbow pain. They further state that decompression of the radial tunnel not only frees the nerve from compression but also relieves tension on the lateral epicondyle and its adjacent structures (Heyse-Moore, 1984). Despite these differences of opinion regarding the prevalence of posterior interosseous nerve entrapment and its causation of lateral elbow pain, the clinical examination process of the injured athlete should include resistive muscle provocation tests and careful accounts of the history and presentation of symptoms.

Another entrapment syndrome that produces pain and disability about the elbow is that of the anterior interosseous nerve. The anterior interosseous nerve arises from the median nerve near the inferior border of the pronator teres. Entrapment of this nerve is reproduced by resisted pronation and often results from activities involving a repetitive screwing motion of the forearm. Weakness of forearm pronation is often accompanied by weak thumb-to-index finger approximation in the involved extremity.

Medial or lateral elbow pain in the presence of distal paresthesias signals the need for additional evaluation of the cervical spine. Although every elbow evaluation should include clearing tests for the cervical spine, intervertebral mobility testing and a full neurological evaluation are recommended when radiculopathy is suspected as the primary cause of distal elbow symptoms.

The evaluative procedures discussed in the next chapter will enable the clinician to rule out differential diagnoses more effectively and better determine the cause and optimal treatment of the athlete with an elbow injury.

CHAPTER 4

Clinical Evaluation of the Elbow

Examination of the elbow requires a comprehensive, sequential, organized approach to determine the localized structure or structures involved and to rule out any related or referral patterns. A thorough understanding of anatomy and biomechanics (see chapter 1), as well as the normal adaptations of the athletic elbow (see chapter 2), enables the clinician to better interpret the evaluation of the elbow. The main components of the clinical examination of the elbow are listed in table 4.1.

TABLE 4.1   Components of the Clinical Examination of the Elbow

Subjective history
Observation/inspection
Palpation
    Bony
    Soft tissue
Related/referral joints (cervical spine, glenohumeral)
Range of motion
    Active/passive
    Endfeel
Accessory movements
Muscular strength testing
Neurological exam
    Reflexes
    Sensation
Special tests

Subjective History

During evaluation of the athlete with an overuse injury of the elbow, basic components of an orthopedic and general medical history should always be included (Gould & Davies, 1985). Specific questions regarding the mechanism of injury should be focused on to better understand the nature and, specifically, the cause of the injury.

As discussed in chapter 1, the throwing motion and tennis strokes can be broken down into stages so as to better understand the forces and muscular requirements inherent in each specific stage. In a retrospective study of 71 throwing athletes with medial elbow instability, 9 percent reported pain during late cocking, 85 percent during acceleration, and 25 percent during follow-through (Conway, Jobe, Glousman, & Pink, 1992). This finding closely matches the description of the valgus stresses imparted to the medial aspect of the elbow in the specific stages of throwing and provides insight into the possible structure(s) involved in the patient being evaluated.

Training history at the time of injury also can be important, due to the fatigue-related nature of many overuse injuries (Leadbetter, 1992). Changes in technique, coaches, and equipment are all of extreme relevance during this portion of the evaluation. Attempts to isolate and localize the injury should be made through specific questions regarding location of symptoms and related/referral history of the cervical spine and shoulder girdle (Dilorenzo, Parkes, & Chmelar, 1990).

Observation/Inspection

Observation of the patient should begin as he or she walks to the evaluation room and during the removal of appropriate clothing. The general posture of the upper extremity is noted, with particular reference to the resting position of the elbow and forearm. If an injury is producing significant intra-articular swelling, the patient will usually hold the elbow in 70° to 80° of flexion, a position that corresponds to the maximum volume of the elbow joint. Obvious deformities in the axial alignment or swelling about the joint should be carefully noted. The elbow normally exhibits a valgus angulation or "carrying angle" of 10° in men and 13° in women (Morrey, 1993). Increases of up to 10° to 15° have been reported in professional baseball pitchers (King et al., 1969).

Swelling or fullness in the lateral recess, just distal to the lateral condyle, indicates an increase in synovial fluid, synovial tissue proliferation, or a radial head pathology. Posteriorly, the olecranon bursa, when inflamed, can produce an obvious deformity from its contents. The degree of muscular hypertrophy or atrophy should be observed in the brachium and forearm, as well as by visual inspection of the posture and musculature of the scapulothoracic region and cervical spine. Elements such as scapular winging and infraspinatus/teres minor muscle atrophy can have significant ramifications for developing a total arm strength treatment program. Weakness of the proximal upper extremity musculature found on initial examination provides an objective rationale for inclusion of exercises that strengthen the entire upper extremity during rehabilitation.

To provide the clinician with an easy reference landmark for determining or approximating the elbow joint line, note that the elbow joint line is located approximately 1 cm below the anterior flexor crease in the antecubital fossa.

Palpation

Palpation of the bony structures about the elbow includes the medial and lateral epicondyles and the olecranon. The relationship between these three bony landmarks is depicted in figure 4.1. In the elbow extension position, the three points normally form a straight line. With flexion of the elbow to 90°, these three landmarks form an isosceles triangle.

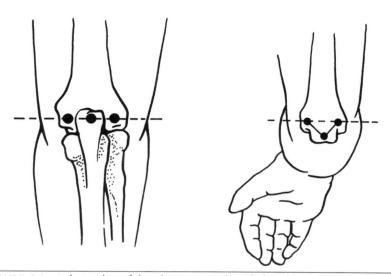

FIGURE 4.1 Relationship of the olecranon and medial and lateral epicondyles forming a straight line in elbow extension (left) and an isosceles triangle in 90° of flexion (right).

Palpation of the bony and soft tissue structures should be performed bilaterally and then compared, similar to other examination procedures. To obtain a baseline, evaluative procedures should be performed on the uninvolved extremity first. Areas the patient describes as tender or sources of extreme pain during the subjective history should be palpated last. According to Clancy (1994), palpation of the most irritable structures first during examination of an injured extremity may cause immediate exacerbation of symptoms. This may overshadow or hide more subtle symptoms present in surrounding tissues that may have been picked up if the primary source of pain had not been elevated by overzealous initial palpation by the examiner.

Bony

The prominent medial epicondyle and attachment of the flexor/pronator muscle can be palpated medially. Proximal to the medial epicondyle is the medial supracondylar ridge, the possible site of osteophytes that can trap the median nerve as well as of the supracondylar lymph nodes. Laterally, the less prominent lateral epicondyle can be palpated, as can the radial head, which is 2 cm distal to the lateral epicondyle. Passive pronation and supination of the forearm will enhance palpation of the radial head. Crepitus and grinding are often present in the radiocapitellar joint due to the lateral compressive forces and bony changes that accompany chronic stress to this region.

Posteriorly, the olecranon can be palpated as a conical bony prominence. With partial elbow flexion and relaxation of the triceps, the olecranon fossa can be palpated. The proximal portion of the ulna both medially and laterally, as well as the subcutaneous aspect of the olecranon, can also be palpated. Continued palpation should be carried out along the posterior aspect of the ulnar border distally to the ulnar styloid. The presence of local tenderness or a bony prominence in the proximal one-third of the ulna may be associated with a stress fracture in throwers (Andrews, Wilk, Satterwhite, & Tedder, 1993).

Soft Tissue

Palpation of the soft tissue structures on the anterior aspect of the elbow in the region of the antecubital fossa includes these structures, from medial to lateral: median nerve, brachial artery, biceps tendon/lacertus fibrosus, and musculocutaneous nerve. The median nerve is not palpable but lies under the brachioradialis muscle as it courses distally. Care should be taken to palpate the distal biceps tendon.

Direct palpation of the distal biceps tendon is warranted in the complete evaluation of the elbow. In an anatomic study, Seiler et al. (1995) found a consistent avascular zone averaging 2.14 cm between a proximal and distal vascular zone within the distal biceps tendon. With the forearm in full pronation, 85 percent of the proximal radioulnar joint space is occupied by the distal biceps tendon. A 50 percent reduction in space in the proximal radioulnar joint due to the radial tuberosity occurs with forearm rotation from supination to pronation. Mechanical impingement, the presence of a hypovascular zone, and high levels of eccentric muscular activity during the acceleration and follow-through phases of the throwing motion and tennis serve can cause tendinous pathology in this region.

Medially, the flexor/pronator muscle group originates on the medial epicondyle. Figure 4.2 shows the positional relationships of the flexor/

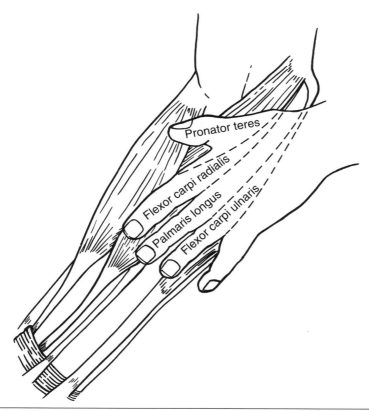

FIGURE 4.2 Anatomical relationship of the flexor/pronator musculature originating on the medial epicondyle of the humerus.

pronator muscles of the medial forearm. Palpation of the ulnar nerve can be performed as it courses under the medial epicondyle in the cubital groove. Bilateral comparison of the nerve with respect to thickness is important. A thickening on palpation of the nerve could signify scar tissue or fibrosis and lead to ulnar nerve compression (Andrews et al., 1993).

The mobility of the ulnar nerve is also assessed. Attempts to dislocate the nerve between the medial epicondyle and olecranon can be assessed and compared bilaterally. Andrews et al. (1993) describes an optimal position for assessment of the mobility of the nerve in the throwing athlete. The supine position is used with 90° of glenohumeral joint abduction and external rotation. The elbow is flexed in a range between 20° and 70° of flexion/extension with palpation of the ulnar nerve and cubital groove.

The medial collateral ligament is difficult to palpate directly. Its course between the anteroinferior surface of the medial epicondyle and the anteromedial ulna can be palpated indirectly for tenderness. In an anatomical study of the flexor/pronator muscle group, Davidson, Pink, Perry, & Jobe (1995) found the flexor carpi ulnaris to be the predominant muscular structure overlying the ulnar collateral ligament (figure 4.2). The flexor carpi ulnaris is the only muscular structure overlying the ulnar collateral ligament during 120° of flexion. The flexor digitorum superficialis is the only other muscle with a close anatomic relationship to the ulnar collateral ligament.

Due to their optimal anatomic location (flexor carpi ulnaris) and relatively large bulk in this region (flexor carpi superficialis), these muscles can ultimately contribute to stability of the elbow and provide support to the ulnar collateral ligament. The anatomic relationship of these muscles to the ulnar collateral ligament is not only relevant when attempting to palpate the ulnar collateral ligament through these muscles, it is also important in rehabilitation of ulnar collateral ligament injury. Ultimate examination of the ulnar collateral ligament is performed with the valgus stress test described later in this chapter.

The posterior soft tissue structures consist mainly of the olecranon bursa and the triceps tendon. The triceps tendon is often tender with direct palpation in cases of posterior tennis elbow.

Laterally, the primary palpable structures include the extensor musculature, which has been termed the mobile wad of three. The "three" consist of the brachioradialis and the extensor carpi radialis longus and brevis. Figure 4.3 shows the positional relationships of the extensor musculature. It is pertinent to reiterate that the extensor carpi radialis longus origin lies proximal to the extensor carpi radialis brevis and just distal to the brachioradialis. The lateral ligamentous structures of the elbow cannot be palpated directly.

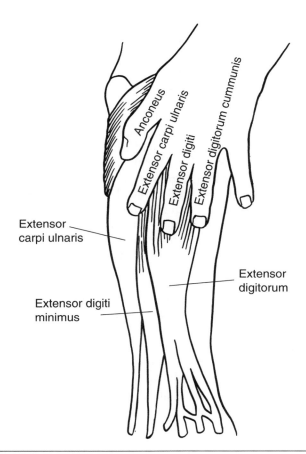

FIGURE 4.3 Positional relationship of the lateral extensor muscles of the forearm. The thumb of the opposite hand overlies the lateral epicondyle along the course of the anconeus, with the other fingers aligning with the course of the extensors of the wrist and fingers.

Related/Referral Joints (Cervical Spine and Glenohumeral Joint)

To further localize and rule out referral symptoms, the joint structures immediately proximal and distal to the injured area must be tested. In addition to evaluating the posture and muscular development of the scapulothoracic region, the cervical spine should be assessed with respect to range of motion in flexion, extension, lateral flexion, and rotation, each with overpressure at end ranges. Localized pain in the cervical spine, and especially radiation of symptoms distally, would warrant a complete evaluation of the cervical spine. Additional assessment of the cervical spine via intervertebral spring testing, particularly in segments referring to the shoulder and elbow (C5-T1), may be necessary if further localization of symptoms is required (Dilorenzo et al., 1990; Gould & Davies, 1985).

Gross screening of the glenohumeral joint is indicated in the evaluation process. Special tests such as the impingement tests of Neer (1973) in forward flexion and Hawkins and Kennedy (1980) in 90° of flexion with internal rotation and cross-arm horizontal adduction are recommended. Evaluation of glenohumeral joint instability in the throwing athlete is also important. Anterior, posterior, and caudal capsular mobility testing in multiple positions of glenohumeral abduction, as well as the load and shift test and subluxation/relocation test of Jobe and Kvitne (1989), should be included to assess the static stability of the glenohumeral joint. Manual muscle testing is also emphasized for the rotator cuff and scapular muscles (Daniels & Worthingham, 1980; Kendall & McCreary, 1983). Nirschl (1977) reports that it is not unusual in evaluating patients with elbow injury to find muscular weakness in the proximal or distal muscle groups on that extremity. Thus, we believe that the inclusion of glenohumeral joint muscular strength testing is of value.

Distally, the wrist is cleared by passive range of motion to end ranges of flexion, extension, and radial and ulnar deviation, with overpressure firmly exerted at end range. Intercarpal joint mobility testing as well as stress applied through the distal radioulnar joint are also assessed and compared bilaterally (Gould & Davies, 1985).

Range of Motion

Assessment of elbow range of motion is an important objective portion of the examination process. Normal joint motion is described as 0° of extension and 145° of flexion (Hoppenfeld, 1976; Kapandji, 1970). Pronation range of motion is normally described as 0° to 85°, with supination range of motion described as 0° to 90° (figure 4.4).

Goniometric documentation of range of motion is recommended to increase the objectivity of the evaluation, and the use of a standardized protocol and universal goniometer has proven reliability for elbow extension/flexion (Fish & Wingate, 1985). Forearm pronation/supination range of motion assessment requires greater care with respect to isolation of proximal movement and is normally measured with the elbow flexed 90° to

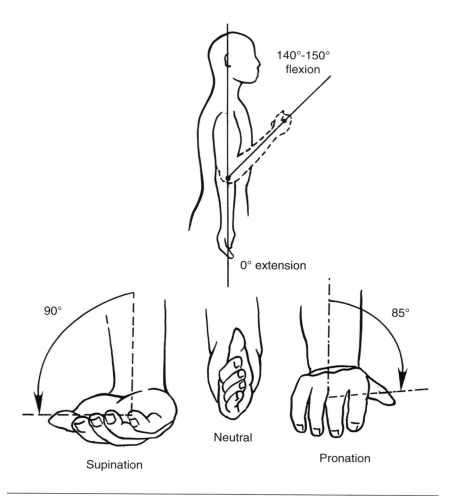

140°-150°
flexion

0° extension

90°

85°

Neutral

Supination

Pronation

FIGURE 4.4   Normal range of motion of the elbow and forearm.

minimize this compensation. Goniometric measurement of wrist extension and flexion with the elbow in the extended position is also warranted because the muscles originating at the elbow span the wrist joint distally. Normal values measured for both wrist flexion and extension are 0° to 85° (Kapandji, 1970).

Hyperextension of the elbow is often seen, particularly in individuals with increased physiological laxity. Assessment of the degree of hypermobility or laxity of an individual's joints includes the gross assessment of elbow hyperextension, genu recurvatum, and metacarpophalangeal joint hyperextension. This gross assessment gives the clinician an overall picture of the individual's relative degree of inherent joint mobility.

Bilateral comparison of range-of-motion measurement is the primary standard for analysis of active and passive range of motion. Passive range of motion of each joint should be checked, as well as the "endfeel." The endfeel is described by Cyriax and Cyriax (1983) as the feeling transmitted to the examiner's hands at the extreme range of passive motion. The normal endfeel of elbow extension is bony, as the olecranon strikes the olecranon fossa (Cyriax & Cyriax, 1983). The endfeel normally associated with elbow flexion is that of soft tissue approximation as the biceps and wrist flexors come into contact with one another. Table 4.2 lists the endfeels described by Cyriax and Cyriax. A capsular endfeel is normally associated with pronation/supination. This capsular endfeel can also be present in the throwing athlete with a flexion contracture for elbow extension. Different endfeels have particular reference to pathology and also form a basis for treatment intensity. For example, an athlete with an empty, painful endfeel is not a candidate for early aggressive strengthening. The endfeel is one aspect of the initial exam that can have direct implications on the initial rehabilitation procedures used.

Accessory Movements

Accessory movements of the elbow are those not under volitional control, but those that occur secondary to the primary movements of elbow extension/flexion and forearm pronation/supination. These accessory movements are abduction/adduction and medial/lateral glide of the ulnohumeral joint, as well as distraction of that joint. The radiocapitellar joint accessory movements consist of compression and distraction as well as ventral and dorsal glides. Again, these movements, similar to the caudal glide of the humeral head within the glenoid with elevation of the shoulder, are not under volitional control.

TABLE 4.2 Classification and Description of Endfeels

Classification	Description
Bony	Two hard surfaces meeting, bone to bone (elbow extension)
Capsular	Leathery feel, further motion available (forearm rotation)
Soft tissue approximation	Soft tissue contact limits further motion (elbow flexion)
Spasm	Muscular spasm limits motion (vibrant twang)
Springy block	Intra-articular block prohibits motion (rebound is felt)
Empty	Movement causes pain, pain limits movement

Accessory movements are assessed bilaterally. Presence of hypermobility of any motion would contraindicate further mobilization of that specific movement. Hypomobility of any of the above-mentioned accessory movements is an indicator for the use of specific joint mobilization techniques during rehabilitation (Bowling & Rockar, 1985). Great care must be taken to avoid overmobilization of the elbow with ligamentous instability; such movement would further jeopardize overall stability and function of the elbow. Further application of the accessory movements of the elbow will be given in chapter 5.

Muscular Strength Testing

Manual assessment of strength, outlined by Kendall and McCreary (1983) and Daniels and Worthingham (1980), is recommended to test the muscular strength of the elbow. Isolation of each muscle is attempted via specific positioning.

To assess brachialis strength, the elbow is flexed with the forearm in a pronated position. Biceps brachii testing is done with the shoulder flexed 45° to 50° and with the forearm supinated. Due to the biceps insertion on the inferior aspect of the radial tuberosity, its peak mechanical efficiency is found with the forearm in a supinated position. The brachioradialis is tested with the forearm in neutral with elbow flexion.

Manual assessment of elbow extensor strength includes the triceps and anconeus, performed with 90° of shoulder and elbow flexion. Pronation/ supination testing should be isolated by using a position of 90° of elbow flexion for testing.

It is important to evaluate the wrist extensors for strength and the provocation of lateral pain. Gross wrist extension testing is not enough when trying to better delineate the injured area. The extensor carpi radialis longus should be tested with approximately 30° of elbow flexion with distal resistance on the base of the second metacarpal, for a combined resistive pattern of extension and radial deviation. The extensor carpi radialis brevis is tested by resisting the base of the third metacarpal with a straight extension force. The extensor carpi ulnaris is tested in a similar extension fashion, with the addition of ulnar deviation to the resistive force (Kendall & McCreary, 1983). Resisted muscle testing is also performed for the extensors with the elbow in complete extension. This places additional tension on the muscle tendon unit and more closely replicates the position of the elbow during particular sport-specific activities. The performance of the muscle with respect to strength and pain during the evaluation is noted and applied to the progression of resistive exercise used during rehabilitation. Testing is also performed for wrist flexion and for gross finger flexion/extension.

Isokinetic evaluation of the elbow is also performed, when applicable, during the initial evaluation of an end-stage injury. Isokinetic testing forms a reliable baseline for the assessment of distal muscular strength at more functional contractile velocities (Davies, 1992). Isokinetic testing and training is discussed at length in chapter 5.

Neurological Exam

Testing the deep tendon reflexes of the distal upper extremity should be performed bilaterally during a thorough evaluation of the elbow complex. The biceps (C5), brachioradialis (C6), and triceps (C7) reflex all have significance when evaluating the injured elbow. Bilateral comparison is essential. Exaggeration of the reflex response may be indicative of an upper motor neuron lesion, with a diminished response indicative of a lower motor neuron lesion.

Sensory evaluation is assessed bilaterally by administering a light touch and determining the patient's subjective responses in each of the areas outlined in Figure 1.7. The regions corresponding to levels C5, C6, C7, C8, and T1 are tested. Diminished sensation over the medial incision following an ulnar nerve transposition or ulnar collateral ligament reconstruction is often reported on the initial postoperative exam. Notation and monitoring of this sensory finding should be part of both the initial and subsequent evaluations of the postoperative elbow.

Special Tests for Examination of the Elbow

Special tests allow for specific testing of the integrity of osseous, ligamentous, tendinous, and neural tissues of the elbow and are an integral part of the complete evaluation of the injured elbow. These tests should be performed and compared bilaterally, with the uninjured extremity tested first.

Tinel's Test

The region of the ulnar nerve overlying the cubital groove is tapped by the examiner's finger, with a positive test producing paresthesias or tingling along the distribution of the ulnar nerve (Morrey, 1993). Tinel's test demonstrates the irritability of regenerating nerve fibers of an injured nerve.

Ulnar (Medial) Collateral Ligament Test

The integrity of the ulnar collateral ligament of the elbow can be tested using a valgus stress test. The test should be administered with the elbow in approximately 25° of flexion. Testing in 25° of flexion removes the olecranon from the olecranon fossa and decreases the bony congruity of the elbow joint, thereby placing greater stress on the ulnar collateral ligament. The extremity being tested should be held such that humeral external rotation is blocked. A valgus stress is exerted while palpating the ulnar collateral ligament region on the medial aspect of the elbow (figure 4.5).

Excessive gaping of the injured extremity, compared bilaterally, indicates attenuation of the ulnar collateral ligament. The amount of opening as well as the perceived endfeel should be noted and compared bilaterally. Pain may be present with the valgus stress applied to the patient's elbow. Isolation of motion to valgus stress without humeral rotation or elbow extension/flexion at the elbow should be targeted.

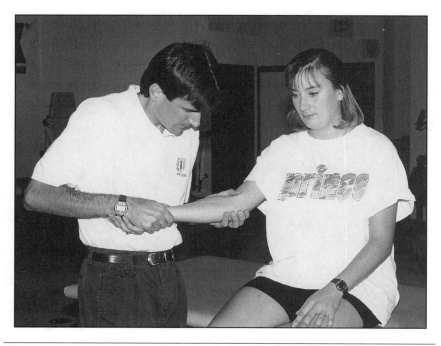

FIGURE 4.5   Valgus stress test for the medial ulnar collateral ligament.

Valgus Extension Overpressure Test

This test has been described extensively by Andrews et al. (1993) to determine whether pain in the elbow is caused by a posteromedial osteophyte abutting the medial margin of the trochlea and olecranon fossa.

The test is performed by extending the elbow while maintaining a valgus stress, simulating the stresses applied during the acceleration phase of the throwing motion or tennis serve. A finger is placed posteriorly along the posteromedial olecranon tip to palpate during the test (figure 4.6). Ten-

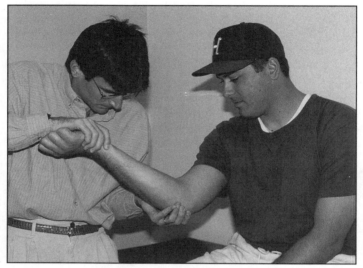

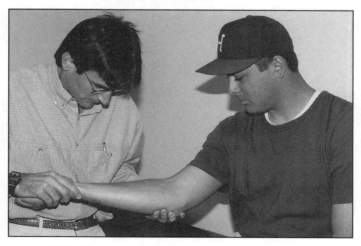

FIGURE 4.6   Valgus extension overpressure test. Starting position (a); a valgus stress is applied by the examiner while extending the elbow (b).

derness, as well as crepitation from an osteophyte or loose body, signifies a positive test. Pain over the posteromedial olecranon is also considered a positive test.

Radiocapitellar Compression Test

The radiocapitellar compression test is initiated with the elbow in extension and one of the examiner's hands cupping the posterior aspect of the elbow with the thumb or index finger over the radial head. The examiner's other hand exerts an axial load to the radiocapitellar joint through the radius via the patient's hand and wrist, the latter of which is held in slight extension and radial deviation (figure 4.7a). Active or passive pronation and supination of the forearm is performed during midrange elbow extension/flexion range of motion while an axial load is applied via the radius. The radial head is palpated during these movements while the radiocapitellar joint is compressed (figure 4.7b). Pain and crepitus in the radiocapitellar joint are indicative of degenerative changes.

Tests for Lateral and Medial Epicondylitis

Tests for lateral epicondylitis involve resistive loading of the extensor musculature during palpation of the wrist extensor common origin (Magee, 1987). Pain in the region of the lateral epicondyle is considered a positive test. Further attempts to isolate the extensor musculature have been discussed previously. Another test described by Magee (1987) for lateral epicondylitis is performed by the examiner as the patient's wrist is first taken into forearm pronation, then fully flexed while the elbow is extended. This test places a tensile stretch on the common extensor tendon and is again positive with pain provocation on the lateral epicondyle.

Similar tests for medial epicondylitis are described using resistive pressure to load the wrist flexors and forearm pronators. Pain in the medial epicondylar region is considered a positive test. Passive placement of the patient's wrist in extension with forearm supination, as well as elbow extension, is also reported (Magee, 1987) as a test for medial epicondylitis.

Elbow Flexion Test

To perform the elbow flexion test, the involved elbow is flexed to end range of motion and held for approximately 5 minutes. This flexed position compresses the ulnar nerve in the cubital groove due to constriction of the cubital tunnel retinaculum and relaxation of the ulnar collateral ligament

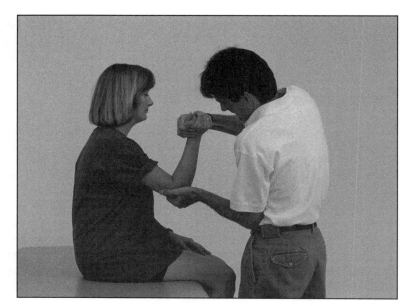

a

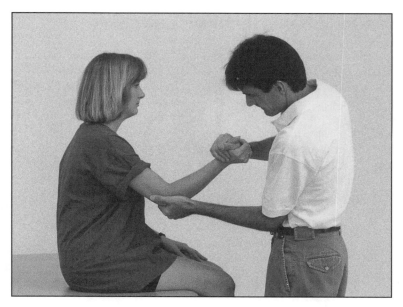

b

FIGURE 4.7   Radiocapitellar compression test. The examiner applies a compressive force along the long axis of the radius via an extended and radially deviated wrist (a). The elbow is then flexed and extended and the forearm pronated and supinated while compressing the radiocapitellar joint (b).

(Morrey, 1993). A positive test is indicated by tingling or paresthesia in the ulnar nerve distribution of the forearm and hand.

"Good Hands" Valgus Stress Test

This test is performed by the patient by placing the ulnar borders of both hands (fifth metacarpals) against each other, with the forearms supinated and elbows in approximately 30° of flexion (figure 4.8). An isometric force is exerted by the patient pressing the ulnar borders of the hands together, keeping them in the "good hands" position. Although this test has not been formally documented, we have used it to test the irritability and sensitivity of the ulnar collateral ligament to light valgus stress. Continued demonstration of this position/maneuver by patients who were throwing athletes, when asked to replicate their symptoms, has led to use of this test in the evaluation procedure. Because the test is performed by the patient, no objective statement regarding instability of the ulnar collateral ligament can be made. The standard valgus stress test is used in conjunction with this maneuver.

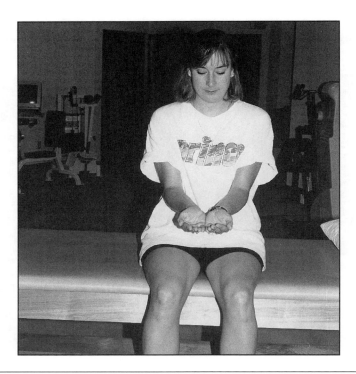

FIGURE 4.8   Good hands test for the medial ulnar collateral ligament complex.

Upper Limb Tension Test (ULTT)

The upper limb tension test is used to determine the presence of adverse mechanical tension (AMT) in the nervous system. AMT in the nervous system refers to multiple entrapment or compression sites of the nervous system affecting overall mobility, specifically the sliding and gliding ability, with response to longitudinal tensioning (Hodges, 1992). The upper limb tension test is believed to be valid for determining the upper limb tension of the neural connective tissue structures (Selvaratnam, Matyas, & Glasgow, 1994).

The upper limb tension test originally described by Elvey (Selvaratnam et al., 1994) attempts to tension the brachial plexus using a combination of upper extremity movements to exert a longitudinal force on the peripheral nerve trunks and cervical nerve roots. The movements of passive shoulder depression, shoulder abduction to 110°, shoulder external rotation and extension behind the coronal plane, forearm supination, and elbow, wrist, and finger extension are components of the upper limb tension test shown in figure 4.9 (Hodges, 1992; Selvaratnam et al., 1994). Cervical lateral flexion away from the limb being tested is also described as a means of further tensioning the nervous system.

An abnormal response to the test may include a decrease in elbow extension range of motion of the injured extremity compared to the contralat-

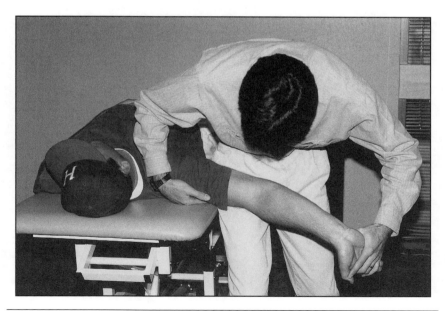

FIGURE 4.9   Upper limb tension test (ULTT).

eral side (Butler, 1994). The normal response to the test position is described as a deep stretch or aching sensation in the cubital fossa extending down to the anterior and radial aspects of the forearm and into the radial side of the hand. A tingling sensation is common in the thumb and first three fingers.

Another version of the upper limb tension test described above is the upper limb tension test 3 (ULTT3), which, unlike other versions of tension testing, involves elbow flexion and is thought to bias the ulnar nerve. Due to the stresses imparted to the medial elbow in throwing athletes, this test variation may also be valuable as an assessment tool.

The components of the ULTT3 include wrist extension, forearm supination, elbow flexion, shoulder girdle depression, and glenohumeral joint external rotation (figure 4.10). The extremity being tested is then brought into glenohumeral joint abduction, maintaining elbow flexion, wrist extension, and forearm supination. The palmar surface of the patient's hand is brought directly toward the ear. The patient's response is again compared bilaterally (Butler, 1994).

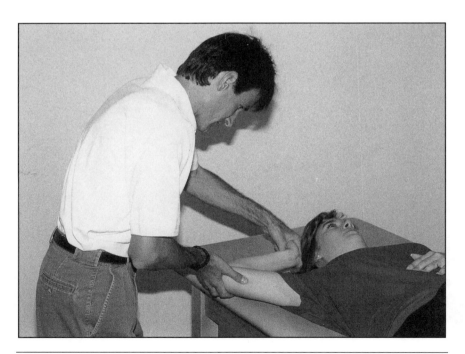

FIGURE 4.10   Upper limb tension test with bias for the ulnar nerve (ULTT3).

CHAPTER 5

Rehabilitation Concepts for the Elbow

The specific rehabilitation approaches to overuse injuries of the elbow presented in chapter 6 rely on an understanding of several key concepts. Integration of these basic concepts following a thorough evaluation is essential to successful treatment and rehabilitation, as well as prevention, of athletic injuries to the elbow.

Regaining Range of Motion

Restoration of normal joint arthrokinematics is a primary goal in the rehabilitation of both nonoperative and postoperative elbow injuries. According to Morrey (1992a), several features of the anatomy of the elbow predispose it to range-of-motion loss and stiffness following injury. These factors include the high degree of congruity and conformity of the ulnohumeral joint, the fact that the joint is traversed by muscle rather than by tendons, and the somewhat unique response of the joint capsule to trauma, resulting in thickening and contracture. These features, coupled with the many descriptive studies that profile racquet sport and throwing athletes reporting flexion contractures as an apparent adaptive response to repetitive activity, often create a clinical challenge during rehabilitation.

The functional arc of motion of the elbow joint for activities of daily living is reported as 30° to 130° of extension/flexion (Morrey, Askew, An, & Chao, 1981). Cooper, Shwedyk, Quanbury, Miller, and Hildebrand (1993) objectively identified both proximal (shoulder) and distal (wrist) joint motion compensation in the presence of limited elbow joint range of motion during ADL activities. A flexion contracture has been reported to place additional stresses on the elbow in throwing athletes (Andrews & Frank, 1985). Several procedures, including stretching and joint mobilization, are used clinically to encourage return of a full range of motion to the athletic elbow and prevent potentially deleterious proximal and distal segment compensations due to a flexion contracture.

Stretching

Early use of the range-of-motion exercises discussed in chapter 6 provide nourishment for articular surfaces and assist in both the synthesis and organization of collagen (Noyes, Mangine, & Barber, 1987; Salter et al., 1980). Active, active-assisted, and passive range of motion of the elbow, forearm, and wrist, as well as the glenohumeral joint, are used extensively to assist in achieving full range of motion of the injured extremity.

In the early phases of rehabilitation, it is important that range-of-motion measures employed by the therapist not be too aggressive. Caution is recommended when pain is present before resistance of motion. In these cases, therapeutic modalities and gentle motion must be used until inflammation and pain are controlled. Overly aggressive range-of-motion procedures are contraindicated early in rehabilitation of the elbow. The relatively thin anterior capsule can be injured easily with aggressive stretching into extension. To further complicate this concept, the brachialis muscle belly traverses the anterior aspect of the elbow joint capsule and actually inserts into the superficial aspect of the capsule. Trauma to the brachialis muscle can cause further scarring and limitation of range of motion. Higher intensity forces applied to the elbow can initiate cellular reactions such as fibroplasia, calcification, and in the most extreme cases, myositis ossificans of the brachialis muscle (Inglis, 1991). Hyperactivity of the stretch reflexes of the triceps and elbow flexors also inhibits range of motion and can interfere with passive stretching techniques attempted during rehabilitation. Therefore, more moderate methods of attaining range of motion are recommended to avoid further scar tissue formation during the initial inflammatory phase of rehabilitation.

Joint Mobilization

Joint mobilization is a widely accepted and recommended practice used by clinicians for restoring normal joint arthrokinematics and full functional ranges of motion (Cyriax & Cyriax, 1983; Kaltenborn, 1980; Maitland, 1970). The application of joint mobilization is based on the assessment of the passive mobility of the ulnohumeral, radiohumeral, and proximal radioulnar joints during evaluation. Use of the grading scale outlined by Kaltenborn

(1980) allows the clinician to categorize the injured segment and determine the appropriate type and intensity of mobilization to use (table 5.1). In many cases following immobilization or subconscious protection of the elbow from injury, the patient will present joint hypomobility, which indicates the inclusion of mobilization in the treatment program. In the case of joint hypermobility, such as with ulnar collateral ligament attenuation, joint mobilization of an already hypermobile segment is strictly contraindicated.

Although a complete discussion of joint mobilization and all its inherent principles is beyond the scope of this text, some principles are worth noting relative to the elbow joint itself.

First, the position of the joint during mobilization has profound implications on effects provided by the technique being applied. The resting position or maximum loose-pack position described by Kaltenborn (1980) is the position in which the joint capsule is most relaxed and the greatest amount of joint play is possible. For the ulnohumeral joint, this position is 70° of flexion with 10° of forearm supination. The humeroradial joint's resting position is in elbow extension with forearm supination, whereas the proximal radioulnar joint's resting position is reported as 35° of supination with 70° of elbow flexion. The resting position is important with respect to mobilization because it provides an optimal reference position for assessing accessory movements. Treatment with mobilization of the elbow is often initiated in this position due to the noncompromising position and interrelationship of the articular structures.

The close-pack position of the joint is the position where maximal tension is present in the joint capsule and ligaments, with maximal contact between the convex and concave articular surfaces (Kaltenborn, 1980). The close-pack position of the ulnohumeral joint is complete extension with forearm supination. The radiohumeral close-pack position is 90° of flexion with 5° of forearm supination. The forearm is in a close-pack position with 5° of supination, the position in which the interosseous membrane is at its tightest. The close-pack position is not used initially in the mobilization sequence because both joint distraction and accessory movements are maximally limited in this position. The close-pack position is

TABLE 5.1   Kaltenborn's Passive Range of Motion Grading Scale

Hypomobility	0 = No movement (ankylosis) 1 = Considerable decrease in movement 2 = Slight decrease in movement
Normal	3 = Normal
Hypermobility	4 = Slight increase in movement 5 = Considerable increase in movement 6 = Complete instability

Data from Kaltenborn 1980.

important to therapists because it affords both maximal stability from joint congruity and ligamentous and capsular tension, and because the joint can be both stabilized and fixed in this position. A joint with inherent instability may be placed in this position for exercise or for treatment other than mobilization due to the enhanced stability inherent in this position.

In addition to the position the joint is placed in during mobilization, the direction of movement is also of importance. The direction of force exerted during mobilization is predicated on the convex/concave theory. When a therapist moves a bone with a convex surface, such as the head of the femur or humerus, the direction of application of the mobilization is in the direction opposite that of the restricted movement. An example of this would be the caudal glide used for treatment of a hypomobile shoulder with subacromial impingement to improve humeral elevation (Ellenbecker & Derscheid, 1989). When a concave joint surface is moved, the direction of application of the mobilization would be the same as the direction of restricted bone movement. The ulnohumeral joint is an example of a concave ulnar joint surface gliding upon the convex distal humerus or trochlea. Therefore, the direction of application of a mobilization technique for the ulnohumeral joint is in the same direction as the restricted movement.

Increasing Elbow Extension

One of the most basic mobilization techniques for the elbow is the use of joint distraction. As with any mobilization technique, the position in which the joint is placed has a drastic effect on the treatment. If joint distraction is applied with the elbow in the resting or loose-pack position (figure 5.1a), structures on both the anterior and posterior aspect of the ulnohumeral joint would be affected equally (Bowling & Rockar, 1985). Placing the elbow in a greater amount of extension with subsequent distraction application would result in a greater stretch to the anterior capsule (figure 5.1b). The normal end range of motion of the elbow joint is limited by tension in the anterior capsule and anterior ligamentous structures, the resistance of the flexor muscles, and the tip of the olecranon entering the olecranon fossa (Kapandji, 1970; Morrey, 1992b). Therefore, mobilization techniques that stress the anterior capsular structures can enhance elbow extension range of motion.

A technique for posterior gliding of the ulna on the humerus is also used to increase extension range of motion. The edge of the treatment plinth or rubber wedge can be used as a fulcrum for the distal aspect of the humerus as the clinician glides the ulna in a posterior direction relative to the humerus (figure 5.2). Again, the amount of elbow extension range of motion used during mobilization dictates the amount of stress imparted to the anterior capsular structures. The 30° angular alignment of the distal

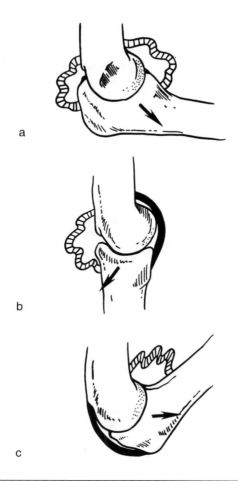

a

b

c

FIGURE 5.1   Medial view of the elbow joint showing distraction in varying degrees of elbow flexion. The degree of stress placed on the capsule based on the joint position used during mobilization is depicted: (a) Resting or loose-pack position. The smooth, solid line seen in (b) and (c) indicates a taut capsule. Arrows show the approximate line of force application by the clinician during mobilization.

humerus and sigmoid notch is an important anatomical relationship for the clinician to understand to ensure proper direction of force application during mobilization.

A medial and lateral glide of the ulna relative to the humerus is reported in the literature as the mobilization of choice to increase overall joint play necessary for full elbow extension range of motion (Kessler & Hertling, 1983). This technique should be used with caution in the throwing athlete and only in the presence of significant joint hypomobility due to possible

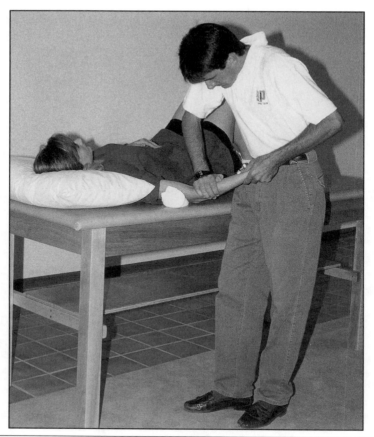

FIGURE 5.2 Posterior glide mobilization of the ulnohumeral joint.

stresses imparted to the ulnar collateral ligament complex. A true medial and lateral gliding motion of the ulna (with the forearm supinated) on the humerus is performed without a varus or valgus movement (figure 5.3). Stabilization of the distal humerus is performed by grasping both humeral epicondyles with the olecranon supported in the palm of the clinician's stabilizing hand. Varying degrees of elbow extension and flexion are recommended, with application of this mobilization technique near the current limits of elbow extension.

Increasing Elbow Flexion

A primary mobilization technique used to increase elbow flexion is joint distraction. With the elbow placed in a position of elbow flexion and forearm supination, joint distraction places greater tension on the posterior

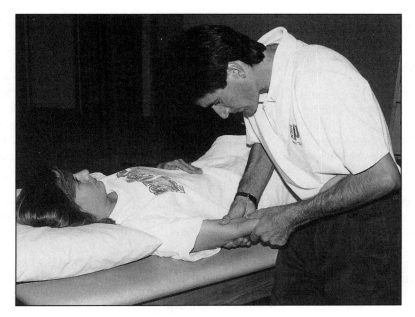

a

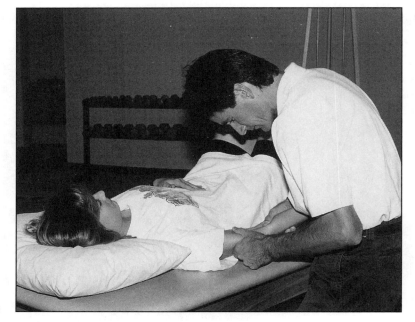

b

FIGURE 5.3 Medial (a) and lateral (b) glide of the ulna relative to the humerus. The stabilizing hand is located proximal to the elbow on the opposite side of the hand directing the force.

capsule (see figure 5.1c). The posterior capsule is one anatomical structure that limits elbow flexion range of motion.

Mobilization of the Proximal Radioulnar Joint

A distal glide of the radius on the ulna, shown in figure 5.4, is used to increase joint play, mainly for reattainment of full elbow flexion and extension. Stabilization of the distal humerus is performed while a long-axis distraction of the radius is achieved by grasping the prominent distal radius. This technique is also considered radiohumeral distraction and is often used in cases of lateral compressive osteochondral injury.

A dorsal/ventral glide of the proximal radioulnar joint is applied to encourage pronation/supination range of motion. The elbow is slightly flexed with the forearm in slight supination. The patient lightly grasps the clinician's arm or waist for support while the clinician glides the radius dorsally and ventrally (figure 5.5).

Again, various positions of forearm pronation/supination and elbow extension/flexion are used for proper stressing of specific structures that can limit forearm motion. It is important for the clinician to realize that the motions of pronation and supination occur due to rotation of the radius around a relatively stationary, stable ulna (Kapandji, 1970). Therefore, because the proximal radioulnar joint consists of a convex radius rotating in

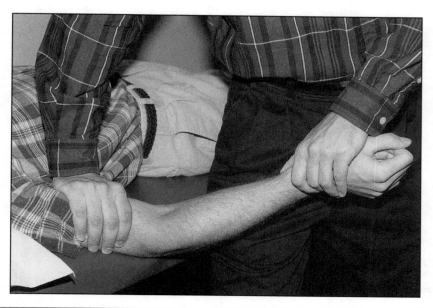

FIGURE 5.4 Distal glide of the radius.

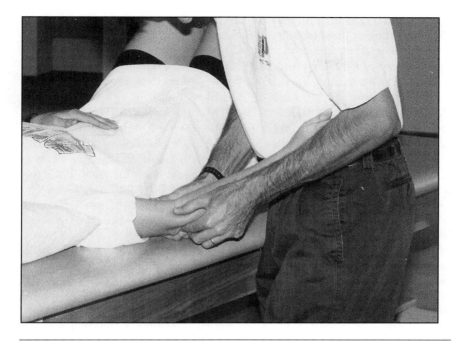

FIGURE 5.5   Dorsal and ventral glide of the proximal radioulnar joint.

the concave lesser sigmoid notch, mobilization of a joint with a convex articular surface moving upon a concave surface results in a direction of application that is opposite the movement restriction (Kaltenborn, 1980). The dorsal and ventral glides of the proximal radioulnar joint can be used to improve pronation/supination range of motion. Based on the convex/concave rule, a ventral glide is applied specifically to increase supination and a dorsal glide is used primarily to increase pronation.

Application of Mobilization and Stretching

The capsular pattern of range-of-motion limitation of the elbow joint describes 10° of elbow extension loss for every 90° of elbow flexion loss (Kaltenborn, 1980). The forearm capsular pattern is described as relatively equal losses of pronation and supination. Application of joint mobilization is based on grades of movement. Kaltenborn and Maitland are the two most commonly cited classifications for grades of movement. Their grading systems are outlined briefly in table 5.2. During the initial inflammatory phase, when pain is the most predominant feature, use of a general joint distraction movement is applied (grade I, Kaltenborn, or grade I with progression to grade II, Maitland). The neutral resting position of the joint (70° of flexion) is used to prevent focal stresses to any one structure. Benefits of low-grade mobilization include pain modulation and joint lubrication (Kaltenborn, 1980; Maitland 1970).

As the inflammation subsides and range of motion limitation and joint stiffness become the predominant clinical features, grades II and III (Kaltenborn) and grades III and IV (Maitland) mobilization are applied. Joint positions progress from the resting, more neutral position to a position at or near end range. Maitland recommends an oscillatory-type movement during application of the specific mobilization technique, whereas Kaltenborn describes a slower, more rhythmical movement held at a terminal point for several seconds (Kaltenborn, 1980; Maitland, 1970). Improvement in range of motion of the accessory movements associated with joint mobilization, such as medial and lateral glides, does produce increases in physiological movement patterns (i.e., elbow extension/flexion) (Kaltenborn, 1980). Additional techniques are applied to encourage range-of-motion attainment in later stages of rehabilitation to complement the joint mobilization procedures outlined here.

Use of a prolonged, low-intensity stretch has produced improvements in elbow extension range of motion. Simple application of a small weight around the patient's wrist has been used to produce a gentle stress into elbow extension (figure 5.6). Care must be taken to avoid using a weight or resistance that is too large. This would elicit pain and a reflex activation or

TABLE 5.2   Grades of Movement

	Kaltenborn	Maitland
Grade I	A small movement in the direction that is done before the performance of a gliding movement—no appreciable joint separation, just enough to nullify joint compression	Small amplitude movement performed at the beginning of the range
Grade II	A movement that takes up the "slack," resulting in tightening of the tissues surrounding the joint	Large amplitude movement performed within the available range, but not reaching the limit of the range
Grade III	A movement taken beyond the "slack," resulting in a stretch of the tissues crossing the joint	Large amplitude movement performed up to the limit of the available range
Grade IV		Small amplitude movement performed at the limit of the range

Data from Kaltenborn 1980 and Maitland 1970.

protective response of the muscle or muscles being stretched and would inhibit the elongation of collagen (Zachazewski & Reischl, 1986).

The contract/relax method can be applied to improve elbow extension range of motion as well. This technique consists of an isometric contraction of the elbow flexors held for several seconds, followed by a relaxation of the elbow flexors and movement of the elbow into extension, either actively or passively. This sequence is repeated, with fatigue of the antagonistic muscle as well as autogenetic inhibitory benefits providing the rationale for use of this technique (Sullivan, Markos, & Minor, 1982).

A low-intensity, long-duration stretch has been reported to produce permanent, plastic deformation of connective tissue (Hepburn & Crivelli, 1984). Plastic deformation of connective tissue refers to a type of elongation where linear deformation produced by tensile stress remains after the stress is removed. This differs from a more elastic deformation in which linear deformation is transient and does not remain following removal of the stress. The goal in range-of-motion enhancement following elbow injury is clearly to achieve a plastic deformation of the connective tissues to allow full extension and flexion. Bonutti, Windau, Ables, and Miller (1994) reported that use of a progressive stretching technique with a long, 30-minute duration

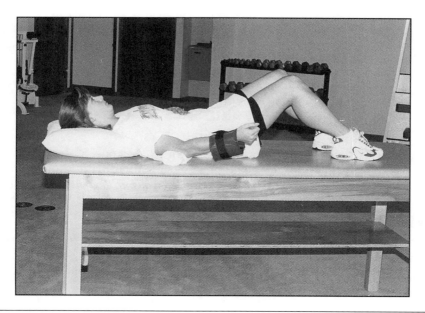

FIGURE 5.6 Low-load/long-duration stretching technique used to increase elbow extension. A towel roll or other wedge is placed proximal to the elbow joint. The use of cuff weights has been found to produce greater relaxation in the patient's extremity than dumbbells, which require a gripping response.

over a one- to three-month interval produced significant increases in elbow extension range of motion in patients who did not respond to other therapeutic techniques for range-of-motion enhancement (including casting and splinting). This prolonged, low-intensity stretching technique is advocated to produce a plastic deformation of the connective tissue.

Summary

The combination of joint mobilization techniques discussed here with early, symptom-predicated, active, active-assisted, and passive range of motion is recommended in rehabilitation of the injured or postoperative elbow. Use of aggressive mobilization or passive stretching early in the inflammatory phases of rehabilitation is severely contraindicated due to the exaggerated scar and reparative properties of the anterior capsule and unique anatomical relationship of the elbow itself. Following the pain/resistance sequence can assist the clinician in determining the appropriate grade of mobilization and level of intensity for stretching during the rehabilitation process (Wilk et al., 1993). Table 5.3 outlines the pain/resistance sequence. Pain before resistance suggests an early inflammatory condition and does not indicate aggressive mobilization or passive stretching. Resistance before pain and a hard or capsular endfeel clearly indicate the use of grade III or IV mobilizations and more aggressive stretching procedures. Specific application of the pain/resistance sequence in clinical rehabilitation of overuse elbow injuries will be discussed in chapter 6.

Isokinetics

Use of the isokinetic mode of resistance is an integral part of the complete rehabilitation and end-stage evaluation of the patient with humeral epicondylitis, osteochondral injury, and both ulnar nerve and ulnar collateral

TABLE 5.3 Pain/Resistance Sequence

Pain before resistance	Acute lesion; active inflammatory response is present—treatment focus on decreasing pain—mild stretching
Pain with resistance	Subacute lesion; mild inflammation present—treatment focus on moderate stretching
Resistance before pain	Chronic lesion; no inflammatory response present—vigorous stretching

Data from Wilk, Arrigo, and Andrews 1993.

ligament injury. The progression of resistive exercise from isometrics to isotonics and eventually isokinetics is followed during rehabilitation. Several important principles regarding isokinetic exercise will provide rationale for the inclusion of isokinetics in elbow rehabilitation.

Isokinetic resistance, initially introduced by Perrine in the 1960s, is characterized by a constant, fixed-velocity, and accommodative resistance throughout the entire range of motion (Davies, 1992). As a joint is taken through a range of motion, the amount of torque that can be produced changes due to the length/tension relationship and changes in the leverage of the musculoskeletal system. Isokinetics can provide an accommodating resistance through the desired range of motion at the desired preset angular velocity. Due to the fast, functional velocities inherent in the distal upper extremity in sport, isokinetic exercise and testing becomes an integral part of the rehabilitation process.

Isokinetic Exercise

In our practice, introduction of isokinetic exercise in the distal upper extremity normally consists of a submaximal trial treatment using speeds ranging from 180° to 300° per second for elite-level athletes and 120° to 180° per second for individuals with lower levels of muscular strength and coordination. Wrist extension/flexion is the initial movement pattern used, with progression to forearm pronation/supination and, finally, elbow extension/flexion in end-stage rehabilitation. This movement pattern sequence has been successful clinically and can promote strengthening of the muscles that cross, and affect, elbow joint function. Use of the wrist flexion/extension and forearm pronation/supination isokinetic movement patterns produces a high level of muscle activation about the elbow with minimal actual elbow joint movement. This maximizes muscular activity but minimizes the stresses imparted to the elbow, as little or no motion is occurring at that joint.

Three to four sets of 15 repetitions are normally performed through the above-mentioned velocity spectrum. A submaximal trial introduction is imperative to prevent patients from exceeding tissue limitations due to the inherent accommodating resistance. Progression to maximal intensity isokinetic exercise is predicated on patient signs and symptoms. A highly repetitive program is normally used, with 15 to 20 repetitions per set for emphasis on the enhancement of local muscular endurance (Fleck & Kraemer, 1987). Rest cycles between sets are customized to the patient's sport activity and energy system demands. A 25- to 30-second rest period is used for tennis players because that is the designated time allowed between points in a tennis match, and rapid recovery following a bout of muscular work is a necessary requirement. According to Fleck (Fleck &

Kraemer, 1987), 75 percent of the adenosine triphosphate (ATP) and phosphocreatine (PC) has been repaid using a 40-second rest period following anaerobic muscular work. A 20-second rest period allows for approximately 50 percent of phosphagen repayment. Therefore, knowledge of both physiological and sport-specific demands of the rehabilitating muscle tendon unit can assist the clinician in the prescription of exercise and determination of rest periods to ensure optimal training parameters for the injured athlete.

The addition of isokinetic exercise to the exercise continuum is ultimately predicated on the individual patient's signs and symptoms and tolerance to resistive exercise during earlier stages of rehabilitation. General guidelines and patterns exist based on postoperative protocols developed from clinical experience with numerous patients. Although significant variation exists, in general, isokinetic exercise is initiated between four and six weeks following arthroscopic elbow surgery. Open surgical procedures of the elbow such as ulnar nerve transpositions and ulnar collateral ligament reconstructions or repair require initiation of isokinetics during more advanced strengthening stages and prior to commencement of an interval throwing program. The normal isokinetic introduction in these cases is between 8 and 12 weeks postoperation. Following the exercise progression from initial isometric and manually resisted exercise to isotonic and then isokinetic exercise provides guidance for inclusion of isokinetic exercise in the rehabilitation program.

Testing and Interpretation

Isokinetic testing of the distal upper extremity produces an objective, reproducible record of the patient's muscular strength (Vanswearingen, 1983). To improve the reliability and validity of the isokinetic test, several training sessions are performed by the patient before maximal isokinetic testing is done (Mawdsley & Knapik, 1982; Wilk, Arrigo, & Andrews, 1991). Five maximal repetitions are used, with peak muscular performance normally measured between the second and fourth repetitions (Arrigo, Wilk, & Andrews, 1994). A consistent, protocol-oriented testing method is recommended by the dynamometer's manufacturer. Attempts to isolate the exercising joint, stabilize adjoining segments to minimize compensation, and anatomically correct interfaces between the patient or subject and the dynamometer are all imperative to ensure quality data generation (Cybex, 1992; Davies, 1992; Wilk et al., 1991). Testing speeds of 90°, 210°, and 300° per second have been used to provide an assessment of strength through the velocity spectrum (Ellenbecker, 1991, 1992b). The order of testing speed begins at 90° and ends at 300° per second. Progressing from the slowest to the fastest isokinetic testing speed has been reported to enhance test-retest reliability (Wilhite, Cohen, & Wilhite, 1992).

Two important parameters used in the interpretation of isokinetic muscle function are peak torque and single-repetition work (Davies, 1992). Peak torque is the highest point on the torque curve regardless of where it occurs in the range of motion. It is indicative of muscular strength at only one point in the range of motion. Single-repetition work is the area under the torque curve and represents muscular strength through the range of motion being tested (Cybex, 1992; Davies, 1992). This parameter is important because muscular strength in both the shortened and lengthened positions is analyzed, as well as in the midrange position, in which the peak torque parameter is often generated. Clinicians use several mechanisms to interpret isokinetic muscle tests. These include bilateral comparisons, normative data comparisons, and unilateral strength ratios.

Bilateral Comparison

One of the most basic methods of interpreting isokinetic muscle tests is through comparison of the injured extremity to the contralateral, uninjured extremity. A descriptive profile of eight professional baseball pitchers undergoing isokinetic wrist extension/flexion and forearm pronation/supination is presented in table 5.4. These patients were evaluated isokinetically a mean of eight weeks following arthroscopy using a Cybex 300 series dynamometer and the testing protocol described earlier.

Results are expressed as the percentage of the injured extremity compared to the uninjured. This is termed a deficit. A negative deficit indicates that the injured extremity's strength actually exceeds that of the uninjured extremity. At eight weeks postarthroscopy, the injured extremities in this sample showed approximately 5 to 10 percent greater strength at speeds of 90° and 210° per second in all four motions tested. Comparisons at 300° per second also showed approximately 25 to 35 percent greater strength for both peak torque and work parameters.

TABLE 5.4 Wrist and Forearm Isokinetic Strength Testing: Average (%) Deficit Peak Torque and Work; Bilateral Comparisons of Eight Professional Baseball Pitchers Eight Weeks Status After Elbow Arthroscopy

Speed	90		210		300	
	Torque	Work	Torque	Work	Torque	Work
Flexion	−3	−1	−3	−2	−14	−14
Extension	−7	4	4	−8	−23	−34
Supination	−6	−13	−7	−16	−25	−28
Pronation	−9	−2	−22	−20	−44	−35

Table 5.5 shows similar comparisons for a sample of 12 professional baseball players following open surgical procedures of the medial elbow (seven ulnar collateral ligament reconstructions and five ulnar nerve transpositions) at a mean of 18 weeks after surgery. The return of muscular strength, particularly in the wrist extensors, flexors, and forearm pronators, is far below that measured in the previous sample following arthroscopic procedures. Although deficits from bilateral comparisons were small following open surgical procedures, significant deficits in muscular strength required for dynamic stabilization of the medial elbow were identified objectively. This finding helps explain why more time is required before interval tennis or throwing programs are initiated following open surgical procedures that expose the medial elbow. More time is required for muscular strength to return to appropriate levels to help protect the underlying ligament and neural structures.

Interpretation of isokinetic testing in the lower extremities is simplified by the fact that lower extremity strength is usually bilaterally symmetrical (Davies, 1992). A dominance effect is an exception, not a normal finding. With the upper extremities, unilateral dominance due to sport or preferential activity may complicate the use of bilateral comparisons. Therefore, normative and descriptive data are a necessary component to ensure that the isokinetic strength test is interpreted properly.

Normative Data for the Distal Upper Extremity

Nirschl and Sobel (1981) initially reported a dominance factor of 5 percent in recreational tennis players and 10 to 15 percent in competitive players based on isokinetic testing of distal muscle groups. Wilk, Arrigo, and Andrews (1993) reported a dominance factor of 10 to 20 percent for the elbow flexors and 5 to 15 percent for the elbow extensors in professional baseball pitchers.

Specific normative data are applied using peak torque/body weight and work/body weight ratios. This creates a relative value of muscular strength

TABLE 5.5 Wrist and Forearm Isokinetic Strength Testing: Average (%) Deficit Peak Torque and Work; Bilateral Comparisons of 12 Professional Baseball Pitchers 18 Weeks Status After Open Surgical Elbow Procedures

Speed	90		210		300	
	Torque	Work	Torque	Work	Torque	Work
Flexion	11	6	0	−6	4	−4
Extension	−2	−3	5	5	2	3
Supination	0	−7	−3	−4	−7	−6
Pronation	−3	−8	−5	−8	−8	−12

for comparison across individuals from a specific population. It is imperative that data from one dynamometer system not be compared to another dynamometer system because of differences in testing position and torque calculation (Francis & Hoobler, 1986).

Data presented in table 5.6 contain a descriptive profile of distal muscular strength of 22 elite tennis players measured on a Cybex II dynamometer (Ellenbecker, 1991). In this population, 10 to 25 percent greater dominant arm strength was found for wrist flexion, extension, and forearm

TABLE 5.6 Peak Torque (PT) and Work (SRW)/Body Weight Ratios in Elite Male Tennis Players Collected on a Cybex II Dynamometer

Motion/speed	Dominant		Nondominant	
	Mean	SD	Mean	SD
Wrist flexion (ft-lb):				
PT 90	14.7	4.8	13.8	3.1
PT 210	13.3	3.4	11.7	3.5
PT 300	11.7	2.7	10.2	2.8
SRW 90	13.4	4.1	12.2	3.1
SRW 210	4.9	1.3	4.3	1.2
SRW 300	2.6	0.7	2.3	0.8
Wrist extension (ft-lb):				
PT 90	10.4	3.3	9.4	2.8
PT 210	8.5	2.2	7.1	2.4
PT 300	7.3	1.9	5.9	1.8
SRW 90	8.5	2.8	7.5	2.5
SRW 210	3.0	0.9	2.4	1.1
SRW 300	1.6	0.5	1.2	0.5
Forearm pronation (ft-lb):				
PT 90	10.1	2.3	8.78	1.9
PT 210	8.0	2.0	6.5	1.7
PT 300	6.7	1.8	5.6	1.9
SRW 90	11.0	3.1	9.4	2.5
SRW 210	3.9	1.2	3.0	0.9
SRW 300	2.1	0.6	1.6	0.6
Forearm supination (ft-lb):				
PT 90	9.3	2.1	8.6	1.7
PT 210	7.1	1.9	6.7	1.7
PT 300	5.5	1.7	5.6	1.7
SRW 90	9.5	2.5	9.1	2.1
SRW 210	3.1	1.1	3.1	0.9
SRW 300	1.5	0.6	1.7	0.6

pronation. No significant difference between extremities was measured for forearm supination strength.

Table 5.7 shows a descriptive profile of isokinetic strength for 10 professional baseball players measured on a Cybex 300 series isokinetic dynamometer (Ellenbecker, 1993). In this elite population, 15 to 35 percent greater wrist flexion and forearm pronation strength was measured, showing specific muscular strength development in these muscle groups. Elbow extension/flexion, wrist extension, and forearm supination did not show significantly greater strength on the dominant extremity.

TABLE 5.7 Peak Torque (PT) and Work (SRW)/Body Weight Ratios in 10 Professional Baseball Pitchers Collected on a Cybex 300 Series Dynamometer

	Arm	
Motion/speed	Dominant	Nondominant
Elbow flexion (ft-lb):		
PT 90	18.9	19.7
PT 210	16.9	17.6
PT 300	15.3	15.5
SRW 90	31.9	35.2
SRW 210	27.1	28.6
SRW 300	21.8	23.5
Elbow extension (ft-lb):		
PT 90	18.4	19.5
PT 210	16.9	17.6
PT 300	15.8	15.9
SRW 90	32.2	34.8
SRW 210	27.5	28.5
SRW 300	27.5	23.6
Wrist flexion (ft-lb):		
PT 90	6.4	5.9
PT 210	5.5	4.8
PT 300	4.8	4.2
SRW 90	7.7	7.3
SRW 210	6.7	5.6
SRW 300	5.9	4.9
Wrist extension (ft-lb):		
PT 90	3.8	4.0
PT 210	3.0	3.1
PT 300	2.7	2.8
SRW 90	4.1	4.4
SRW 210	3.4	3.5
SRW 300	2.9	2.8

(continued)

TABLE 5.7   *(continued)*

Forearm pronation (ft-lb):		
PT 90	5.0	4.2
PT 210	4.4	3.3
PT 300	3.7	2.6
SRW 90	7.1	5.9
SRW 210	6.4	4.8
SRW 300	5.7	4.1
Forearm supination (ft-lb):		
PT 90	4.0	4.1
PT 210	3.3	3.3
PT 300	2.9	2.8
SRW 90	5.5	6.0
SRW 210	4.9	4.9
SRW 300	4.6	4.6

Data from isokinetic research provide information for determining the degree of unilateral dominance in athletes using the upper extremity extensively. In addition, strength scores from both the dominant and nondominant extremity can be compared to the population-specific data presented here. This allows for further analysis of postinjury or postoperative distal strength for a more scientific and objectively oriented determination of both the patient's progress and muscular status. Returning the elite athlete with unilaterally dominant upper extremity strength to only equal bilateral strength may not be acceptable rehabilitation, whereas returning a nonathletic individual to a level of symmetrical upper extremity strength may be all that is required.

Unilateral Strength Ratios (Agonist/Antagonist)

In addition to bilateral and normative data comparisons, assessment of the balance of muscular strength is also essential. The unilateral strength ratio is produced by dividing the weaker muscle group into the corresponding parameter of the opposing muscle group. Table 5.8 contains the unilateral strength ratios measured in 22 elite tennis players. The wrist extensors are only 60 to 70 percent as strong as the wrist flexors in this population. Forearm supination strength is 75 to 80 percent of forearm pronation strength.

Table 5.9 shows the unilateral strength ratios for professional baseball pitchers. Slightly higher extension/flexion ratios are reported in elite tennis players compared to the sample of baseball pitchers. This is to be expected based on the high levels of wrist extensor muscle activity during tennis-specific movement patterns (Morris et al., 1989).

TABLE 5.8   Unilateral Peak Torque (PT) and Work Strength Ratios (SRW) for the Distal Upper Extremity of Elite Male Tennis Players Collected on a Cybex II Dynamometer

	Arm	
Ratio/speed	Dominant	Nondominant
Wrist extension/flexion (%):		
PT 90	71	68
PT 210	64	61
PT 300	63	58
Mean	66	62
SRW 90	64	61
SRW 210	61	57
SRW 300	62	55
Mean	62	58
Forearm supination/pronation (%):		
PT 90	93	98
PT 210	88	104
PT 300	83	101
Mean	88	101
SRW 90	86	97
SRW 210	80	103
SRW 300	75	103
Mean	80	101

Use of the unilateral strength ratio for rehabilitation and preventive isokinetic screening yields important information regarding muscular balance. One important factor in rehabilitation of the athlete using the upper extremity extensively is normalization of muscular balance. The selective, adaptive development of upper extremity muscle groups warrants careful analysis and specific exercise prescription to ensure proper balance of muscle function surrounding the joints.

Balancing the external/internal rotation ratio in the shoulder is a prime example of the important relationship between muscular imbalance and pathology. Warner, Micheli, Arslanian, Kennedy, & Kennedy (1990) found consistent alterations of the normal unilateral external/internal rotation ratios in patients diagnosed with glenohumeral impingement and instability. Imbalances of the unilateral external/internal rotation ratio have been reported in the dominant shoulders of elite tennis players (Chandler, Kibler, Stracener, Ziegler, & Pace, 1992; Ellenbecker, 1991, 1992b). Additionally, the unilateral external/internal rotation ratios of the dominant shoulder of elite tennis players were found to have a significant statistical relationship to serving velocity (Cohen et al., 1994).

TABLE 5.9   Unilateral Peak Torque (PT) and Work Strength Ratios (SRW) for the Distal Upper Extremity of Professional Baseball Pitchers Collected on a Cybex 300 Series Dynamometer

Ratio/speed	Arm	
	Dominant	Nondominant
Elbow flexion/extension (%):		
PT 90	103	101
PT 210	100	100
PT 300	97	98
SRW 90	100	101
SRW 210	99	100
SRW 300	99	100
Wrist extension/flexion (%):		
PT 90	59	67
PT 210	54	64
PT 300	56	64
SRW 90	53	60
SRW 210	51	63
SRW 300	49	57
Forearm supination/pronation (%):		
PT 90	80	98
PT 210	75	100
PT 300	78	107
SRW 90	77	101
SRW 210	77	102
SRW 300	80	112

Carryover of this concept to the distal upper extremity can be seen in athletes with exaggerated wrist flexion and forearm pronation muscular strength ratios. The important eccentric function of the muscle groups (wrist extensors and forearm supinators) opposing the hypertrophied muscles (wrist flexors and forearm pronators) is necessary to produce normal mechanics and controlled movement patterns (Glousman et al., 1992). Additionally, the supinator muscle's close association with the lateral ligament complex (annular ligament) may also provide dynamic ligament tension and vital stabilization to the joint.

Summary

Isokinetic assessment of muscular strength is one important aspect in the clinical decision to progress the patient to an interval functional return program. Criteria for this return include functional joint range of motion, absence of pain on direct palpation and during clinical examination, and strength levels acceptable for the activity level of the patient. For example, bilaterally symmetrical strength is normally required in elite-level athletes prior to commencement of an interval return program because eventually 20 to 30 percent greater strength is required. A recreational athlete often begins the early, submaximal stages of a cautious interval program with 10 to 15 percent strength deficits.

Bilateral comparison, normative data, and unilateral strength ratios are all used to provide objective guidance for clinical progression of the patient during rehabilitation. Identification of areas for continued emphasis in a home exercise program, as well as exercise recommendations for preventive conditioning, can be objectively predicated on isokinetic tests of muscular strength.

The Total Arm Strength Concept

Both rehabilitation and prevention of an overuse injury in the upper extremity require a comprehensive approach. Inherent in that approach are a thorough evaluation to determine the pathomechanics of injury and the baseline strength and flexibility of the athlete. Due to the complex interaction of the individual segments of the upper extremity with activities of daily living or composite athletic movement patterns, a program addressing the entire upper extremity kinetic chain is required for both rehabilitation and prevention of elbow and shoulder injury.

The upper extremity kinetic chain comprises the musculature and articulations of the trunk, scapulothoracic, scapulohumeral, and distal arm segments (Davies, 1992). This concept is predicated on the work of Hanavan (1964), who created a mathematical representation of the human body consisting of conical links comprising the lower and upper extremities and trunk. In reference to upper extremity skill performance, work in these segments is transmitted to the trunk and spine through a large musculoskeletal surface; this results in the production of massive amounts of energy, with each joint in the kinetic chain cumulatively adding its load and serving as a fulcrum for proximal and distal segments. Schmier (1945) states that the strength with which a segment of the body moves also depends on the synergistic response of distant muscles, which, by their action, do not even move the segment being tested. The application of these concepts forms the primary rationale for using a total arm strength approach in both rehabilitation and preventive conditioning programs in athletes.

Use of the total arm strength concept with respect to rehabilitation of overuse elbow injuries is detailed in chapter 6. The repeated use of proximal glenohumeral and scapulothoracic muscular strengthening techniques and closed-chain exercises promoting proximal co-contraction in the upper extremity is highly recommended for the prevention of upper extremity injury as well. Weakness in the upper extremity kinetic chain has been identified in recreational tennis players with tennis elbow through measurement of composite upper extremity strength when compared to healthy tennis players and a healthy control group (Strizak, Gleim, Sapega, & Nicholas, 1983). The detailed anatomical descriptions of muscular, osseous, and vascular upper extremity adaptations were identified in the review of descriptive profiles of the upper extremities of baseball and tennis players in chapter 2.

The Kinetic Link Principle

Treatment and prevention of overuse injuries in the upper extremity also involve the application of the kinetic link principle. The use of biomechanically optimal mechanics for throwing or tennis requires integration of the kinetic link principle to enhance performance and especially prevent injuries. The kinetic link principle provides the framework for the description of optimal mechanics via power generation to the upper extremity by the larger, more powerful muscles of the lower extremity and trunk (Groppel, 1992; Kibler, 1994). To prevent overload to smaller muscles of the shoulder and elbow, the primary sources of power generation should be derived from both linear and angular momentum of the trunk and lower extremities. Use of proper trunk and shoulder rotation during the throwing motion and tennis strokes provides essential energy for proper execution and protection.

One extremely important element in the prevention of elbow injuries in the overhead-motion athlete is the adherence to proper mechanical execution of the throwing, tennis serve, or tennis groundstroke motions. This is an important part of the final rehabilitative process and is closely monitored by execution and evaluation of the interval sport performance program under direct observation in the clinic.

Throwing

Although many individual variations exist in the throwing motions of elite players, several characteristic similarities found during biomechanical research are normally used to promote optimal throwing mechanics. In a clinical study correlating injury to the method of delivery used in the throwing motion, Albright, Jokl, Shaw, and Albright (1978) found three primary factors in the mechanics of pitchers with arm injury: (1) opening the lead shoulder prematurely, which leaves the dominant shoulder and elbow to drag behind the rest of the body; (2) extension of the glove hand; and (3) lifting the back foot from the mound too soon.

Opening the lead shoulder prematurely also contributes to increasing stress on the anterior aspect of the shoulder, as well as increasing tensile load on the medial elbow (Albright et al., 1978). The second two factors outlined by Albright and colleagues point to the important interaction of segments far from the injured shoulder or elbow as playing a direct part in injury. The legs and contralateral limb provide significant energy transfer to the throwing arm; when these segmental interactions become uncoordinated, injury can ensue.

In addition to these factors, biomechanical study of the throwing arm shows a relatively consistent trunk-to-arm alignment of 90° at the glenohumeral joint (Fleisig et al., 1989). This position is consistent regardless of the style of delivery, such as sidearm or overhand. The degree of lateral flexion of the trunk does change to give the appearance of a different point of release based on the delivery style of the pitcher. Deviation from this 90° angle at the shoulder could have grave consequences, especially if the shoulder is placed in a greater degree of abduction. This would place the shoulder in a potential position of impingement and increase the tension on the ligamentous structures of the anterior and inferior aspect of the shoulder. Likewise, the degree of flexion of the elbow can change the amount of stress placed on the capsuloligamentous structures of the medial elbow.

An & Morrey (1993) profiled the changing loads on the medial ligaments based on the degree of flexion/extension of the ulnohumeral joint (see Table 1.1, page 8). Inappropriate elbow position during the late cocking and acceleration phases of the throwing motion, such as increased elbow flexion (often termed short-arming the ball), can be a compensation used by the throwing athlete to protect the shoulder following injury to or surgery on the glenohumeral joint. Consequently, throwing with the elbow in a more extended position creates a longer lever arm at the glenohumeral joint and can negatively affect the shoulder and elbow.

Finally, one other finding in the throwing motion that can lead to increased stress on the elbow is cupping the ball by excessively flexing the wrist as the throwing hand and ball are released from the glove early in the cocking phase. This maneuver requires a greater range of motion and more muscle activity to achieve a position of wrist extension later in the cocking phase (Perry & Glousman, 1990).

Inappropriate execution of the curveball and other breaking pitches by excessive forearm and wrist activation has also been reported by many patients being evaluated with elbow pain. This has been especially true in the prepubescent and adolescent populations who have open physes, substandard distal muscle strength and endurance, and poor coordination. We recommend learning the proper biomechanical sequences under the direct supervision of a biomechanist or coach as an integral part of the total rehabilitation and preventive program.

Tennis Serve and Groundstrokes

Similar to the precise biomechanical interactions of the kinetic chain in throwing, the tennis serve and groundstrokes also require optimal mechanics to prevent injury and optimize performance. The position of the elbow during impact of both the forehand and backhand uses the osseous, ligamentous, and dynamic muscular stability to prevent focal stresses to the structures surrounding the elbow (Groppel, 1992; Nirschl & Sobel, 1981). The most common biomechanical characteristic reported in the literature as a causative factor in lateral epicondylitis is the leading-elbow backhand (Bernhang et al., 1974; Groppel, 1992; Nirschl, 1977; Nirschl & Sobel, 1981). The leading-elbow backhand places the elbow in a position of increased flexion and causes greater activation of the extensor muscles of the wrist (Kelley et al., 1994). Additionally, lateral elbow symptoms can also be caused by excessive forearm pronation on the tennis serve or forehand (Ellenbecker, 1995). Attempting to produce topspin using inappropriate forearm pronation during the forehand can increase the stress imparted to both the medial and lateral structures at the elbow. The decelerative activity of the forearm supinators required following concentric pronation can increase the stress on the lateral muscle tendon structures.

To support the important concept of emphasizing use of proper mechanics for the prevention of overuse elbow injuries, Ilfeld (1992) studied the mechanics of 57 patients with tennis elbow. Success rates ranging from 82 percent in chronic cases to 90 percent in acute cases were reported with conservative treatment and professional instruction to improve the stroke or strokes that led to manifestation of the injury.

CHAPTER 6

Treatment and Rehabilitation of Overuse Elbow Injuries

Treatment of the injured elbow involves specific, systematic evaluation and rehabilitation methods to address the deficiencies or pathology identified. This chapter presents approaches to initial management of the injured elbow, followed by an extensive review of the specific rehabilitation methods used for elbow injuries.

Immediate Management

Immediate management of the patient with an overuse injury of the elbow begins with basic principles of acute injury care. Protection of the elbow and surrounding structures is mandated without necessarily resting the elbow from complete function in all cases. Protection from further injurious stress is important; however, complete immobilization is not always indicated due to the possibility of disuse atrophy occurring in muscular structures that are already weakened and broken down from overuse (Leadbetter, 1992; Nirschl & Sobel, 1981). Initial goals are to decrease the inflammation and pain response, prevent contractures through promotion of available joint range of motion, and when appropriate, use submaximal exercise to retard muscular atrophy.

The immediate management of the injured elbow, as outlined above, contains two critical elements. The first is to begin measures to decrease pain and inflammation in the injured structures using ice, gentle compression, and protection of the injured elbow from further stress. The second is to obtain the necessary initial evaluation measures that lead to a complete diagnosis of the injury. As a physical therapist or athletic trainer, this means referral of the patient to an appropriate physician to obtain a comprehensive medical evaluation, including x-rays and other diagnostic procedures, if necessary. Nonsteroidal anti-inflammatory medication is often prescribed to assist in diminution of the inflammatory condition (Kamien, 1990; Rosenthal, 1984). Following the initial medical evaluation, nonoperative evaluation and rehabilitative measures are begun.

Humeral (Lateral and Medial) Epicondylitis

Initial treatment of the patient with humeral epicondylitis involves nonoperative rehabilitation (Nirschl, 1977; Nirschl & Sobel, 1981). According to Nirschl (1992), 92 percent of the humeral epicondylitis cases evaluated responded favorably to nonoperative treatment. Consistent with other overuse injuries of the elbow, surgical or operative management is applied only after an extensive course of nonoperative treatment fails.

Nonoperative Treatment and Rehabilitation

There are four stages or phases of nonoperative rehabilitation of humeral epicondylitis:

- Reduction of overload, pain, and inflammation
- Promotion of total arm strength and normal joint arthrokinematics
- Interval return to full activity, and
- Maintenance

Progression of the patient through these phases forms the primary treatment program for the successful nonoperative rehabilitation of humeral epicondylitis.

Phase I: Reduction of Overload, Pain, and Inflammation

Modalities.   Consistent reports in the literature regarding treatment of humeral epicondylitis involve the initial stage of treatment of this syndrome. The reduction of pain and inflammation in the muscle/tendon unit is imperative before other significant range-of-motion or strengthening procedures are employed. Although many published reports agree on the initial goal in treatment, significant variation in treatment methodology exists. The use of ultrasound (Bernhang et al., 1974; Nirschl & Sobel, 1981), electric stimulation and ice, cortisone injection (Kamien, 1990; Nirschl & Sobel, 1981), nonsteroidal anti-inflammatory medication (Rosenthal, 1984), acupuncture (Brattberg, 1983), transverse friction massage (Ingham, 1981), and dimethyl sulfoxide (DMSO) application (Percy & Carson, 1981) have all been reported in the literature.

The treatment methodologies have been studied in comparative analyses to determine their effectiveness. A retrospective study of 70 patients with lateral epicondylitis by Dijs et al. (1990) found the greatest initial relief of symptoms from cortisone injection (91 percent short-term improvement) compared to 47 percent from traditional physical therapy. The most notable result from this study is the incidence of recurrence with the two treatment methods studied. Cortisone injection treatment had a 51 percent recurrence rate after three months, whereas the recurrence rate with physical therapy was only 5 percent. Kivi (1982) compared the effects of two types of injections (cortisone and methylprednisone) with an immobilizer and anti-inflammatory medication. No significant difference was found among the three methods tested. Stratford, Levy, Gauldie, Miseferi, and Levy (1989) evaluated the effects of phonophoresis, ultrasound with placebo, and friction massage and found no significant difference among groups.

Analysis of the literature comparing treatment modalities does not indicate a single, most effective choice. Labelle et al. (1992) reviewed 185 articles on the treatment of humeral epicondylitis and found glaring defects in the scientific quality of the research investigations. Further research, using both blind and random testing methodologies, must be done to identify scientifically and clinically the optimal method or methods for decreasing the initial pain and inflammation associated with humeral epicondylitis. Therefore, considerable clinical differences continue to exist in the initial treatment of humeral epicondylitis.

Using guidelines set forth in earlier literature, we normally use treatment modalities consisting of ice, electrical stimulation, ultrasound, phonophoresis, and iontophoresis. Clinical experience has not identified a particular treatment or treatment sequence that is more effective than any other in the initial diminution of pain and inflammation. Consistent use of ice following early attempts at exercise or unavoidable ADL activities by the patient during the initial stages of rehabilitation is greatly emphasized. Repeated use of therapeutic modalities is applied during the initial phase of treatment, with gradual weaning of the patient as signs and symptoms allow.

The region of modality application is generally directly over the most affected areas subjectively reported by the patient, as well as any area of palpable tenderness documented during the initial examination. Common sites of localized tenderness are shown in figure 6.1.

In a review of 70 patients with tennis elbow, Dijs et al. (1990) reported the incidence of maximal tenderness corresponding to the locations described

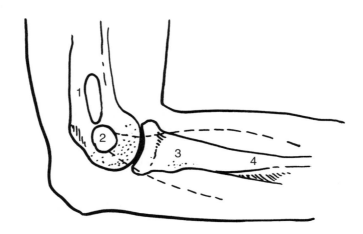

FIGURE 6.1   Common sites of localized pain in patients with lateral epicondylitis: (1) origin of extensor carpi radialis longus, (2) origin of extensor carpi radialis brevis (ECRB), (3) tendinitis of the muscle tendon junction of the ECRB, and (4) strain of the muscle ECRB.

in figure 6.1. They reported incidences of 1, 90, 1, and 8 percent, respectively. These results are consistent with our clinical findings of maximal localized tenderness over the origin of the extensor carpi radialis brevis tendon in patients with lateral humeral epicondylitis. In patients with medial epicondylitis, the most common sites of tenderness and subsequent modality treatment administration are the common flexor/pronator tendon on the medial epicondyle and the flexor/pronator muscle tendon junction.

If there is lack of progress with initial modality application over a period of two to three weeks, the patient should return to the referring physician for further evaluation and possible cortisone injection. Clinical signs that indicate the ineffectiveness of therapeutic modalities are (1) continued pain at rest or with light activity, (2) inability to tolerate light stretching/range-of-motion exercise, and (3) continued inability to perform submaximal exercises to increase strength. These signs not only convey a lack of patient progress but are a concern because of the patient's inability to perform early range-of-motion or strength exercises that ultimately are required to return normal function to the injured area.

Immobilization/bracing.   Immobilization should be applied cautiously during the early phase of rehabilitation, according to Nirschl (1977, 1992; Nirschl & Sobel, 1981). One approach is to use a wrist immobilizer, which indirectly protects the elbow by limiting wrist movement, hence affording rest to the extensor and flexor muscle groups that cross the elbow. Coonrad and Hooper (1973) advocate the use of a dorsiflexion splint for early treatment of humeral epicondylitis.

We have used the wrist immobilizer in a limited, short-term application during the initial stages of rehabilitation. The immobilizer appears to also serve as a mechanical reminder to the patient that the extremity is injured and encourages use of the uninjured, often nonpreferred extremity. Due to the negative effects of further disuse atrophy in muscles with already compromised levels of strength and endurance (Leadbetter, 1992; Nirschl, 1992), care must be taken in global distribution of the immobilizer either in a patient population that is not being monitored by a therapeutic exercise program or for long duration of use.

Strengthening.   Early submaximal exercise is begun as signs and symptoms allow. Nirschl (1977) uses patient tolerance to a firm handshake as a criterion for determining whether a patient is ready for early exercise in the treatment program. We advocate early use of submaximal isometrics and manual resistive exercise. It is important to note that even though symptoms exist in either the lateral or medial epicondyle, early submaximal resistance exercise can be initiated in the unaffected muscle groups. For lateral epicondylitis, exercise is recommended for the flexors and pronators, in addition to the obvious work required by the extensors and supinators to prevent disuse atrophy and normalize distal muscle function. The Cybex upper body ergometer (UBE) (Cybex, Inc., Ronkonkoma, NY) is also used early in rehabilitation because of its noncompromising range of motion and promotion of total arm (both proximal and distal) muscular work (figure 6.2).

The initial goal of rehabilitation, with respect to the muscle tendon unit, is the promotion of muscular endurance and improved resistance to repetitive stress (Nirschl & Sobel, 1981). To accomplish this goal, extremely low or no resistance is used with high-repetition formats of 25 to 45 per set. This promotes local muscular endurance and provides a vascular response to the exercising tissues as well (Fleck & Kraemer, 1987).

Range of motion.   Integration of range of motion and general upper extremity flexibility is gradually performed during the initial stage of rehabilitation. Aggressive end-range passive stretching and mobilization are not indicated, due to the potential deleterious effects on the muscle tendon unit. Maintenance of pain-free elbow, forearm, wrist, and finger motion is the goal in this phase.

It is important to remember the presence of flexion contractures on the dominant arm in the throwing or racquet sport athlete frequently reported in the literature. In most cases, acute or even chronic humeral epicondylitis does not produce flexion contractures caused by degenerative changes in

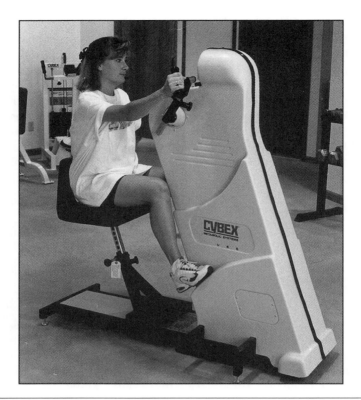

FIGURE 6.2   Upper body ergometer (UBE). (Cybex, Inc., Ronkonkoma, NY)

the tendon. The flexion contracture measured during the initial examination of the throwing or racquet sport athlete is generally an adaptation to the repetitive demands of specific sport activities (Chinn et al., 1974). Thus, aggressive end-range mobilization in the elbow with humeral epicondylitis is not generally indicated, especially in early phases of rehabilitation. Comfortable range of motion and stretching of the elbow, forearm, and wrist musculature are used during this phase. Additionally, stretching of the musculature about the shoulder is applied to prevent range-of-motion loss in the proximal structures, especially during the period of either activity modification or rest.

Phase II: Promotion of Total Arm Strength and Normal Joint Arthrokinematics

Range of motion.   As inflammation and pain levels in the injured area decrease, greater emphasis is placed on range of motion and muscular strength and endurance. As previously mentioned, we do not advocate aggressive stretching during the initial phases of rehabilitation of the patient with humeral epicondylitis. However, if the injured elbow exhibits significant range-of-motion limitation relative to the uninjured elbow, joint distraction and mobilization to enhance ulnohumeral extension are recommended during this phase. These techniques are discussed on pages 66-68. In most cases of overuse injury, only active-assisted and passive stretching of the elbow, forearm, and wrist using intensities well tolerated by the patient (far below pain and reflex activation levels) are necessary to return normal, bilaterally symmetrical motion to the injured extremity.

As described in chapter 2, the dominant elbow in athletes with a unilaterally dominant upper extremity often contains a flexion contracture that has not developed acutely but from repetitive stress and compensation. Clinical judgment must be exercised by the treating clinician as to the degree of emphasis and potential for range-of-motion enhancement on an individual basis.

We use the endfeel classifications described by Cyriax and Cyriax (1983) (see table 4.2) as one key indicator of that potential. A bony endfeel does not indicate potential for range of motion improvement, whereas a more capsular or muscular spasm endfeel does indicate potential for range-of-motion improvement with joint mobilization and modality therapies. An empty endfeel should warn the clinician to be cautious regarding the use of stretching and mobilization techniques at end range due to the inflammatory implications that correspond to the empty endfeel (Cyriax & Cyriax, 1983).

In addition to elbow flexion contractures, Ellenbecker (1992a) reported significant wrist extension range-of-motion deficits in elite junior tennis players measured with a standard universal goniometer. Tightness in the flexor/pronator muscle group limiting wrist extension range of motion with the forearm in a supinated position is a common initial evaluation finding in the patient with an overuse elbow injury. This finding supports the use of stretching of the elbow, forearm, and wrist when treating athletes in this population.

Active-assisted and passive stretching, using several repetitions and hold durations of 15 to 30 seconds, are indicated to attempt to produce a plastic deformation of the muscle tendon unit (Zachazewski & Reischl, 1986). A supine patient position is recommended to enhance the clinician's ability to perform combined patterns of elbow, forearm, wrist, and finger movements relative to the glenohumeral joint and trunk. Knowledge of the combined upper extremity kinetic chain movement patterns (see chapter 1) enables the clinician to appropriately stress the extremity in preparation for eventual return to the demands of the athlete's sport.

Resistive exercise.   Progression of resistive exercise from the initial stage of isometrics and manual resistance is recommended during the second

WRIST STRENGTHENING EXERCISES

- Never work through specific elbow joint pain.
- Avoid jerking; work slowly through the range of motion.
- Begin with three sets of 10 and progress to five sets of 10 unless otherwise instructed.
- It is very important to slowly lower or return the weight to the starting position to emphasize an eccentric or lengthening contraction.

Wrist Curls (Extensors)

Sit in a chair with elbow flexed and forearm resting on a table or over your knee with the wrist and hand hanging over the edge. The hand is turned so the palm is down. Stabilize the forearm with the opposite hand and slowly curl your wrist and hand upward. Be sure to move only at your wrist, not at your elbow. Raise hand slowly, hold for a count, and slowly lower weight. Repeat.

Wrist Curls (Flexors)

Sit in a chair with elbow flexed and forearm resting on a table or over your knee with the wrist and hand hanging over the edge. The hand is turned so the palm is up. Stabilize the forearm with the opposite hand and slowly curl your wrist and hand upward. Be sure to move only at your wrist, not at your elbow. Raise hand slowly, hold for a count, and slowly lower weight. Repeat.

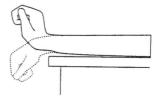

Forearm Rotation (Pronation/Supination)

Sit in a chair with elbow flexed and forearm resting on a table or your knee with the wrist and hand hanging over the edge. Using a dumbbell with weight at only one end (e.g., a hammer), begin the exercise with the palm-up position (A). Slowly raise the weight by rotating your forearm and wrist to the upright position (B). Hold for a count and slowly return to the starting position (A). When finished with the recommended number

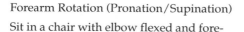

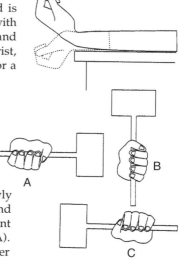

of repetitions of this exercise, begin the exercise again in the palm-down position (C). Slowly raise the weight by rotating your forearm and wrist to the upright position (B). Hold for a count and slowly return to the starting position (C). Repeat.

Radial Deviation

In a standing position with your arm at your side, grasp a dumbbell with weight on only one end. The weighted end should be in front of your exercising hand. With your forearm in the neutral position (thumb pointing straight ahead of you), slowly raise and lower the weight through a comfortable range of motion. All the movement should occur at your wrist with NO elbow or shoulder joint movement. You will not be able to exercise through a very large arc of movement. Repeat.

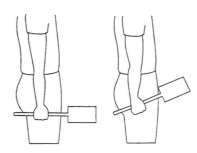

Ulnar Deviation

In a standing position with your arm at your side, grasp a dumbbell with weight on only one end. The weighted end should be behind your exercising hand. With your forearm in the neutral position (thumb pointing straight ahead of you), slowly raise and lower the weight through a comfortable range of motion. All the movement should occur at your wrist with NO elbow or shoulder joint movement. You will be able to exercise through a relatively large arc of movement. Repeat.

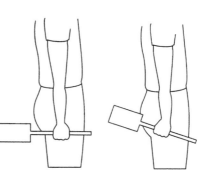

Grip Strengthening

Begin with elbow bent 90° at your side. Place a tennis ball or putty in the palm of your hand. Squeeze firmly; hold for 3-5 seconds. Release pressure. Repeat until fatigue occurs. As pain allows, progress to performing this exercise with the elbow straight.

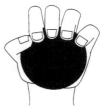

phase. The modes of resistive exercise followed in the rehabilitation of overuse injuries are

- multiple-angle isometrics,
- manual resistance isotonics,
- isotonics (concentric and eccentric emphasis), and
- isokinetics.

This progression of resistive exercise is outlined extensively by Davies (1985) for rehabilitation of the muscle-tendon unit.

Isotonic concentric and eccentric exercise using the movement patterns listed under "Wrist Strengthening Exercises" on pages 96-97 are used. Modification of these exercises is often necessary initially due to intolerance of the patient to performing the exercises with the elbow in complete extension. Modifying the exercises to an elbow flexed position places the muscles that cross the elbow in a more shortened position. The patient should progress to full elbow extension during these exercises because many sport-specific movement patterns involve muscular control at near-terminal elbow extension (Groppel, 1992; Kibler, 1994; Werner et al., 1993).

Initial isolated submaximal eccentric contractions of the wrist extensors for lateral epicondylitis, and of the wrist flexors for medial epicondylitis, are used if the patient is unable to perform the exercise movement pattern concentrically against gravity. The eccentric mode of isotonic exercise is used initially due to the higher internally generated muscle tensions and force production hierarchy (Elftman principle) inherent with eccentric muscle work (Davies & Ellenbecker, 1992; Doss & Karpovich, 1965; Komi & Buskirk, 1972). A low-resistance, high-repetition format is used to increase not only strength but local muscular endurance as well.

Performance of the resistive exercises is predicated on the response of the patient. Localized pain in the insertional region of the tendon on either the medial or lateral epicondyle is not accepted. Exercise intensities must be regulated such that a pain-free range of motion and pain-free resistance level are used at all times during rehabilitation. A feeling of muscular fatigue or tightness is accepted as a normal, productive response from the patient.

Integration of both concentric and eccentric phases of the distal upper extremity isotonic exercises is emphasized through a slow, controlled movement pattern by the patient throughout the duration of exercise. Free weights and surgical tubing are both employed during this phase of rehabilitation. Six weeks, three times per week, of wrist extension/flexion training with surgical tubing using three sets of 10 repetitions in healthy, uninjured subjects did not produce significant strength improvements measured before and after training on an isokinetic dynamometer (Ellenbecker, Kingma, & Kim, 1994). Despite this finding among healthy uninjured subjects, we believe that low to moderate levels of concentric and eccentric resistance provided by surgical tubing and free weights with a high-rep-etition format should be an integral part of the rehabilitation process for overuse injuries in the athletic elbow.

Proprioceptive neuromuscular facilitation (PNF) diagonal patterns, es-pecially diagonal 1 (flexion), which involves scapular abduction, upward rotation, and elevation, shoulder flexion, adduction, and external rotation, elbow flexion, and wrist flexion and radial deviation, and diagonal 1 (ex-tension), which includes scapular depression, adduction, and downward rotation, shoulder extension, abduction, and internal rotation, elbow ex-tension, and wrist extension and ulnar deviation, are used during this phase to promote neuromuscular control (Sullivan et al., 1982). The use of rhyth-mic stabilization and slow reversal holds is emphasized, particularly for the extremity distal to the ulnohumeral joint.

Consistent with the total arm strength concept of phase II, strengthen-ing exercises for the proximal aspect of the upper extremity kinetic chain are added during this phase. The isolated rotator cuff strengthening pro-gram listed in "Shoulder Strengthening Exercises" on page 100 is started to promote proximal muscular strength and muscular balance. As reported by Nirschl (1977), manually assessed strength deficits in the rotator cuff are often associated with humeral epicondylitis.

The exercises shown on page 100 are based on EMG research of the muscles surrounding the glenohumeral joint and elicit high levels of rota-tor cuff activation (Ballantyne et al., 1993; Blackburn, McLeod, White, Wofford, 1990; Townsend et al., 1992). Both concentric and eccentric mus-cular work are emphasized through slow, controlled execution of these exercise movement patterns. Use of these exercises is delayed if their per-formance has negative effects on the origin of discomfort in the elbow. In clinical observation, we have found that these proximal rotator cuff exer-cises seldom exacerbate distal symptoms.

Additional exercises using low resistance levels and multiple repetitions are employed during this phase of rehabilitation. Scapular exercises, includ-ing the seated row and manual protraction/retraction resistance, are also recommended (Moseley et al., 1992). Surgical tubing is used for concentric and eccentric muscular strengthening of the elbow flexors (using varied po-sitions of forearm rotation) and elbow extensors (triceps and anconeus).

Exercises involving the upper extremity in a closed-chain state (distal member of the extremity fixed during exercise) are also employed during this phase. The extremity is placed so that the elbow is in a comfortably extended position over a large, inflatable ball, with the extremity bearing progressive amounts of weight into the ball. As with any closed-chain ex-ercise, this position causes co-contraction of the musculature surrounding multiple joints via multiple joint axes (Palmitier, An, Scott, & Chao, 1991). Clockwise and counterclockwise circles of various sizes are performed by the patient, as well as crosslike patterns and diagonals.

SHOULDER STRENGTHENING EXERCISES

Sidelying External Rotation

Lie on uninvolved side, with involved arm at side and a small pillow between arm and body. Keeping elbow of involved arm bent and fixed to side, raise arm into external rotation. Slowly lower to starting position and repeat.

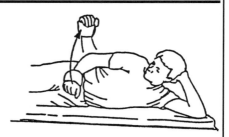

Shoulder Extension

Lie on table on stomach with involved arm hanging straight toward the floor. With thumb pointed outward, raise arm straight back into extension toward your hip. Slowly lower arm and repeat.

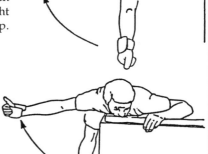

Prone Horizontal Abduction

Lie on table on stomach with involved arm hanging straight toward the floor. With thumb pointed outward, raise arm out to the side, parallel to the floor. Slowly lower arm and repeat.

Supraspinatus—"Empty Can"

Stand with elbow straight and thumb pointed down toward the ground. Raise arm to shoulder level at 30° angle to body. Slowly lower arm and repeat.

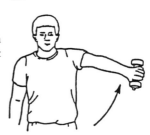

90/90 External Rotation

Lie on table on stomach with shoulder abducted to 90° and arm supported on table with elbow bent at 90°. Keeping the shoulder and elbow fixed, rotate arm into external rotation; slowly lower to start position and repeat.

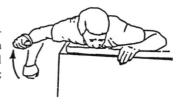

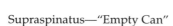

Figure 6.3 shows an example of a closed-chain exercise using an inflatable therapy ball. A handgrip platform (OPTP, Minneapolis, MN) is used to interface the patient's extremity to the ball. Without the platform, the wrist is placed in a hyperextended position pressing against the ball, which can cause secondary discomfort. The inflatable therapeutic ball is also used in the rhythmic dribbling exercise shown in figure 6.4. Small, rapid dribbling movements are performed for 30- to 60-second durations, progressing from ground to eye level, with 120° of shoulder flexion.

The BOING (OPTP, Minneapolis, MN) is another tool used to exercise the distal upper extremity. Various oscillatory patterns are used, including wrist and elbow extension/flexion, forearm pronation/supination, and radial/ulnar deviation (figure 6.5). Again, durations of this exercise favor the development of local muscular endurance and vary from 30 to 60 seconds per set.

Once a functional range of motion in the wrist and elbow is achieved and patient tolerance to the isotonic exercises has been demonstrated, the patient is progressed to isokinetic exercise. For both lateral and medial

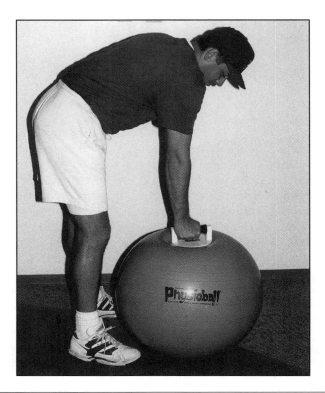

FIGURE 6.3   Closed-chain exercise using a therapeutic ball.

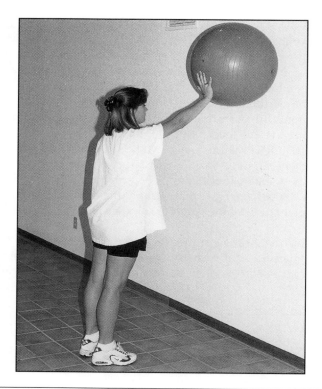

FIGURE 6.4   Rhythmic dribbling exercise using a therapeutic ball with the shoulder in approximately 120° of elevation.

humeral epicondylitis, a submaximal trial treatment in the pattern of wrist extension/flexion is used. The elbow is placed in 60° to 90° of elbow flexion during initial training, as shown in figure 6.6. Isokinetic speeds of 180° to 300° per second have been used for the trial treatment, with sets and repetitions starting with as few as three sets of 15 repetitions. Progression to five to six sets of 15 to 20 repetitions is commonly employed in later stages of rehabilitation using the velocity spectrum between 180° and 300° per second. Emphasis on use of a high-repetition program continues with the isokinetic mode of resistance for enhancement of local muscular endurance. Progression of forearm position using isokinetic dynamometers is recommended. For lateral humeral epicondylitis, a forearm-supinated position is used initially, with progression as tolerated to a forearm-pronated position, due not only to the functional characteristics of this position but also to the need to exercise the weaker wrist extensor muscle group against gravity.

Isokinetic exercise training in the movement pattern of forearm pronation/supination is added once the patient demonstrates a tolerance to the

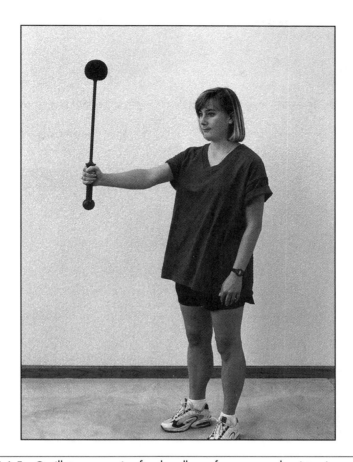

FIGURE 6.5 Oscillatory exercise for the elbow, forearm, and wrist using a BOING device. Stabilization and co-contraction of the distal and proximal upper extremity musculature are required to oscillate the device as shown. Multiple movement patterns can be executed.

wrist extension/flexion position. The elbow is placed in approximately 60° to 90° of elbow flexion during exercise, as pictured in figure 6.7, with progression in later stages of rehabilitation to a position with greater degrees of elbow extension, due to the more extended position inherent in many upper extremity sport activities (Ellenbecker, 1992a).

The use of plyometric exercises is recommended in the later stages of the total arm strength phase of rehabilitation. These exercises are characterized by an eccentric or lengthening contraction of a muscle followed immediately by a concentric or shortening contraction of the same muscle. The time it takes to reverse the direction of a plyometric exercise (between the eccentric and concentric contractions) is termed the amortization phase

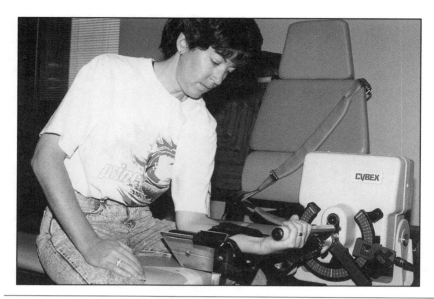

FIGURE 6.6   Isokinetic wrist extension/flexion setup on a Cybex isokinetic dynamometer system.

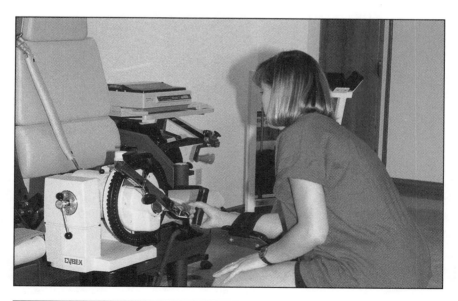

FIGURE 6.7   Isokinetic forearm pronation/supination setup on a Cybex isokinetic dynamometer system.

(Chu, 1989). The concept or principle behind plyometric exercise is that stretching of the series elastic components of the muscle and activation of the stretch reflex from the eccentric muscular contraction during the lengthening phase of the exercise enhances the subsequent concentric or shortening response of the muscle. This process is also termed the stretch-shortening cycle (Wilk & Arrigo, 1993).

During the later stages of elbow rehabilitation, plyometric exercises are applied using medicine balls and the Plyoback system (Functionally Integrated Technology, San Marcos, CA). Weighted Plyo-Balls weighing from as little as 2 pounds to 6 to 9 pounds are used in typical patterns such as the standard basketball chest pass and overhead double-handed soccer throw. Figure 6.8 shows the two-handed chest pass and the Plyoback system.

Variations on the standard chest passes are an alternating two-handed forehand and backhand stroke simulation pass, the sideways shoulder throw (figure 6.9), as well as a simulated throwing movement with the shoulder in 90° of abduction with 90° of elbow flexion (figure 6.10). With the arm in the 90/90 position, isolated internal and external rotation of the shoulder with a 2-pound medicine ball creates a valgus stress on the medial elbow structures. The adaptive stresses used in this exercise prepare the elbow for the inherent valgus stresses placed on the medial aspect of the elbow in throwing or serving. The forearm pronators and wrist flexors must stabilize the medial aspect of the elbow as the shoulder is brought

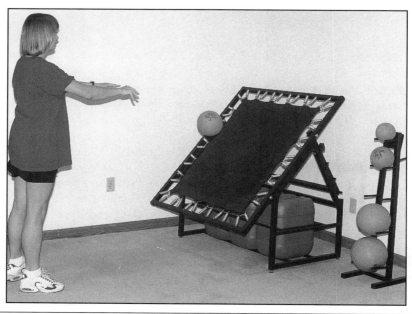

FIGURE 6.8   Plyometric chest pass exercise using the Plyoback system.

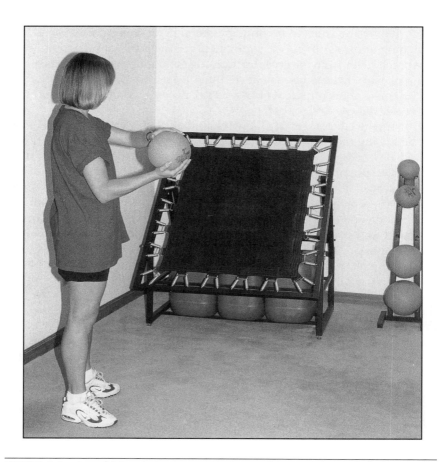

FIGURE 6.9   An additional plyometric exercise used to stress the medial elbow in the later stages of rehabilitation. The sideways shoulder throw is used in a diagonal cross-body pattern, as shown.

into external rotation with 90° of elbow flexion during the eccentric loading phase of the exercise.

As with all upper extremity plyometric exercises, the amount of time the ball is held is minimized by encouraging the patient to catch and release the ball as quickly as possible to emphasize the rapid, explosive muscular work inherent in plyometric exercise. Therapeutic gym physioballs can also be used initially if the weight of commonly available medicine balls is too great. The rapid accelerative and decelerative movements inherent in plyometric exercise make it an integral part of preparing the injured segment for functional activities.

Finally, isokinetic elbow extension/flexion training (figure 6.11) is applied following patient tolerance to wrist extension/flexion and forearm

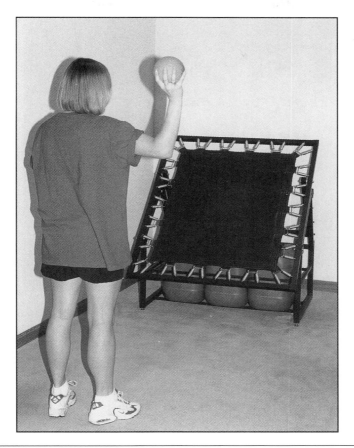

FIGURE 6.10   Plyometric exercise in 90/90 position with the Plyoback system.

pronation/supination isokinetic training patterns. Further discussion regarding the use of isokinetics in rehabilitation of the elbow, including interpretation of test results and the use of normative data, can be found in chapter 5.

Heavy reliance on home exercise programs is necessary to continue the patient's progression of resistive exercise. The distal upper extremity exercises presented on page 100 are given to the patient to provide additional exercise at home using light weights or surgical tubing. Because clinical exercise time is often limited and local, distally oriented exercise takes priority; thus, the rotator cuff and scapular program is often performed at home or on days without actual clinical rehabilitation. Care must be taken not to overexercise the patient at too early a stage in rehabilitation, and the initial limitation of home involvement may be necessary, particularly in the highly motivated or overzealous individual.

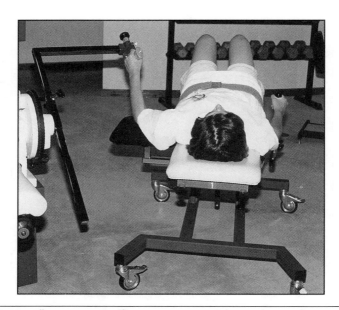

FIGURE 6.11   Elbow extension/flexion setup on a Cybex isokinetic dynamometer system.

During rehabilitation, and especially with preparation for the return to activity following humeral epicondylitis, control and reduction of overload forces are vital to the comprehensive rehabilitation process. External bracing, equipment modification, and functional activity analysis and alteration are critical parts of this process.

Counterforce brace.   The external arm support or brace used to decrease overload forces is the counterforce brace recommended extensively by Nirschl (1977, 1992), Nirschl & Sobel (1981), and Groppel & Nirschl (1986). This brace consists of a 2- to 2.5-inch-wide nonelastic strap (figure 6.12) with Velcro fasteners used to prevent full muscular expansion (two fasteners are preferred by Nirschl due to the conical nature of the proximal forearm) (Froimson, 1971).

Limitation of full muscular expansion by the nonelastic brace should decrease the force generated by the muscle itself and reduce stress on the tendinous insertion on the epicondyle. Nirschl theorized the brace's clinical effectiveness and positive biomechanical alteration based on EMG activity of the wrist extensor muscles during tennis play via decreasing and diffusing the affected muscles' internally generated contractile tension (Groppel & Nirschl, 1986). Snyder-Mackler and Epler (1989) also reported a reduction in the EMG activity of the wrist extensors with an Aircast tennis elbow counterforce brace compared to control values. Inconsistent strength relationships have been reported by Anderson and Rutt (1992)

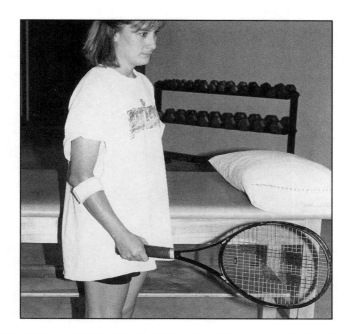

FIGURE 6.12 Counterforce brace applied for reduction of overload for lateral epi-condylitis.

and Stonecipher and Catlin (1984) using isokinetic testing of the forearm and wrist with and without a counterforce brace in normal subjects. Further research is necessary to quantify objectively the effect of counterforce application on muscular strength.

Limited, early use of the wrist immobilizer is replaced by the counterforce brace for activities of daily living that require heavy forearm use such as typing, writing, or driving. Continued use of the counterforce brace is recommended during the interval sport return program and for several months following a full return to athletic participation.

Equipment Evaluation and Modification.   Evaluation of the patient's equipment is also important prior to beginning an interval return tennis program. No definitive relationship between tennis elbow and racquet head size, stiffness, and balance has been identified, although a causal relationship between these factors and the forces exerted on the elbow is reported throughout the literature (Bernhang et al., 1974; Groppel, 1992; Nirschl, 1977, 1992; Nirschl & Sobel, 1981). Nirschl recommends a midsize racquet of medium flexibility for patients with tennis elbow (Nirschl, 1992).

Evaluation of the patient's tennis racquet has several important areas of emphasis. Most modern racquets come in a midsize (90- to 95-square-inch racquet face) and oversize (110-square-inch) frame. An oversize racquet

HYPEREXTENSION ELBOW BRACE

A neoprene sleeve to protect the elbow from hyperextension and valgus stress during throwing and other functional activities has been developed by Todd Ellenbecker and Rick Dehart, ATC and is available through Joint Solutions (Tustin, CA). The brace has been used during the return-to-activity phase of rehabilitation following ulnar collateral ligament injury and ulnar nerve transposition. In addition to preventing end-range extension of the elbow, the medial and lateral hinges placed within the neoprene sleeve can provide protection against valgus stresses incurred with throwing.

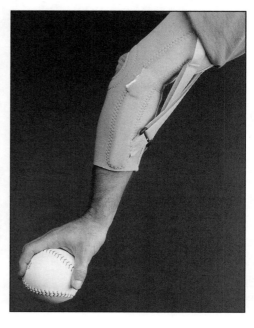

will generate more power and provide greater vibration dampening than an identical frame with a midsize racquet face (Groppel, 1992). Racquet stiffness is of major concern to the player's extremity. Modern frames are wider (widebody frame classification) and have greater inherent stiffness to produce greater power and also dampen vibration. The stiffer the racquet, the less forgiveness there is on off-center impacts and the greater the shock or jar transmitted to the arm (Roetert, Brody, Dillman, Groppel, & Schultheis, 1995). Therefore, a more flexible racquet will soften the feeling of initial impact and may be indicated for patients with upper extremity overuse injuries. With respect to racquet weight, most sports medicine professionals recommend a light to medium-light frame that is evenly balanced or head light to enhance maneuverability and optimize stroke preparation and proper mechanics (Nirschl, 1992).

Another important aspect of equipment evaluation is how the tennis racquet is strung. Contrary to what most novice tennis players and the

TENNIS RACQUET TECHNOLOGY

The most notable recent change in racquet technology has been the "widebody" tennis racquet. The desire to provide a stiffer tennis racquet has led to use of materials such as graph-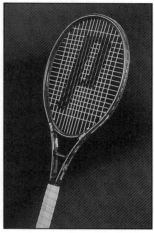ite, Kevlar, and boron in racquet manufacturing. To further stiffen the racquet, design changes were made by increasing the width of the racquet frame. Also affecting the stiffness of the frame is the shape of the racquet. The smoother the transition from the widest to narrowest part of the racquet cross section, the stiffer the racquet will be (Groppel, 1992). This principle allows racquet manufacturers to manipulate the stiffness of the frame locally, in the racquet head or shaft. As a result, nearly every racquet manufacturer has developed a series of widebody tennis racquets.

A stiffer racquet will provide greater power because the shaft bends less in response to impact, thus less energy from the incoming ball velocity is lost. A stiffer racquet frame will dampen out vibrations more quickly because it is vibrating at a higher frequency, but a greater amount of shock or jarring is imparted to the arm with this stiffer, widebody design (Roetert et al., 1995).

Although a direct relationship between a particular type of racquet and injury has not been systematically reported, the increased stiffness of the racquet frame, especially with the initial change to a stiffer racquet by a tennis player, does produce a risk of overuse injury similar to a runner changing to a new type of shoe or altering his or her training program. Additionally, the frame itself may not cause injury, but the compensatory muscle activity patterns often dictated by the stiffer, more powerful tennis racquet to control this power can result in injury. Inappropriate attempts to generate topspin to control the powerful postimpact ball velocities generated by a stiffer frame may cause elbow or shoulder injuries, as discussed previously.

Although technological advances continue to provide greater evaluative insight for the clinician, improvements in technology that allow more powerful and skillful sports performance can also effect injuries to the athletic elbow. Continued research in sports medicine and science is necessary to give the clinician a greater understanding of the demands on and requirements of the elbow in sport-specific activities.

general public believe, research indicates that a lower string tension creates greater postimpact ball velocity and hence produces greater power with lower stroke effort from the player. A higher string tension gives greater control to the racquet and produces a lower postimpact ball velocity compared to the same racquet strung more loosely. It is often recommended that players restring their racquet with a few pounds less tension when returning to play following an upper extremity overuse injury (Ellenbecker, 1995; Groppel, 1992; Nirschl, 1977, 1992; Nirschl & Sobel, 1981; Roetert et al., 1995).

Various devices made of foam or numerous densities of plastic or rubber are commonly placed between the strings of the tennis racquet to decrease vibration. Brody (1989) studied the vibration-dampening characteristics of such devices and found them effective for diminution of high-frequency string vibration but not for lower frequency, more damaging frame vibration. Although these devices are effective at quieting string vibration postimpact, no positive effect on the upper extremity can be attributed to them. Kuessner (1991) reported that vibrations from the racquet that may cause injury are transmitted through the racquet head itself.

The grip of the racquet is also important with respect to optimizing performance. Proper grip size can be estimated using the Nirschl technique, demonstrated in figure 6.13. A ruler is used to measure from the tip of the ring finger to the proximal palmar crease. When choosing between a smaller or larger handle size, the larger is usually preferred, as less effort is required merely to hang onto the racquet (Groppel, 1992). Research monitoring EMG activity of the anterior deltoid and wrist extensors with different racquet handle sizes does suggest lower activity levels in the forearm extensors on the backhand groundstroke with a larger racquet handle (Adelsberg, 1986).

Even elite players do not strike the ball directly in the most optimal racquet location on every impact, and with novice players, off-center and off-axis impacts are a frequent occurrence. All of the tennis racquet characteristics mentioned have some effect on these types of impacts as well. The hand and arm twist along the long axis of the racquet regardless of how tightly it is gripped. A racquet with torsional flexibility and softer, looser strings results in the angular impulse being spread out over a slightly longer time, reducing the abruptness and harshness of the interaction (Roetert et al., 1995).

Another factor related to racquet grip is the degree of tightness with which the racquet is held during play. Most highly skilled players grip the racquet in a submaximal fashion through most of the groundstroke cycle, increasing grip firmness just prior to impact, indicating an efficiency or economy with respect to repetitive wrist extensor muscle activity (Nirschl, 1984). Many novice players have a "deathgrip"-type racquet/hand interface, which results in stiffness of the wrist and early muscular fatigue of

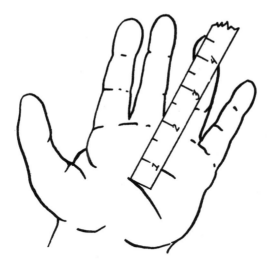

FIGURE 6.13   Tennis racquet grip sizing method recommended by Nirschl (1977). A ruler is used to measure the distance from the tip of the ring finger to the proximal palmar crease.

the forearm. Grabiner, Groppel, & Campbell, (1983) found no significant difference in postimpact ball velocity with two extremes of grip firmness. Gripping the racquet in a firm manner rather than a "deathgrip" is recommended by tennis teaching professionals.

Modification of equipment for activities other than tennis is also recommended. Increasing the handle size on hammers and screwdrivers, as well as increasing the length of screwdrivers, can improve the mechanical advantage and leverage (Nirschl, 1977). Differing shafts or handles on hammers and other tools can be manipulated to change the stiffness and relative forgiveness during repetitive impacts. No significant difference in EMG activity of the wrist flexors was found with manipulation of golf club grip size in subjects suffering with medial epicondylitis (Glazebrook et al., 1994). Although this study found no significant difference, the authors concluded that further study must be done with regard to equipment modification and muscular activity patterns.

Activity Analysis and Alteration.   Activity analysis and alteration are an important part of the interval return programs outlined later in this chapter. During an interval return program, the patient's stroke mechanics or throwing motion are evaluated and modified on a regular basis with video analysis, if available. A three-dimensional video analysis can provide extensive information to both the clinician and researcher; however, simple performance of patient activity on video, captured from multiple perspectives, can greatly assist the clinician and, most important, often provide feedback to the athlete regarding his or her mechanics.

Phase III: Interval Return to Full Activity

Evaluation of the patient for a return to full activity includes specific assessment of upper extremity range of motion and strength. A full, pain-free range of motion in the elbow, forearm, and wrist is required before the patient can be considered an optimal candidate for return to full activity. Assessment of strength using isokinetics, if available, or manual muscle testing is also recommended in the comprehensive evaluation. Appropriate levels of strength compared bilaterally, as well as normal balance of the unilateral muscle ratios, are expected before a functional return is recommended (see discussion on the use of isokinetics in rehabilitation of the elbow in chapter 5). A handgrip dynamometer is also used as a gross strength measure for bilateral comparison. Typically, an athlete with a unilaterally dominant upper extremity will have a minimum of 10 percent and up to 25 to 30 percent greater grip strength on the dominant arm compared to the nondominant extremity (Ellenbecker, 1991; Nirschl & Sobel, 1981). We place greater emphasis on isokinetic test results as opposed to either handgrip dynamometers or manual assessment, because of the dynamic nature of the isokinetic test and degree of objectivity (Davies, 1992; Ellenbecker, 1992a).

Interval tennis return program.   The interval tennis program we developed is presented in Appendix B, Interval Return Programs: Tennis. An extremely important part of the rehabilitative process is reemphasis on proper sport mechanics. This emphasis has been present from the initial evaluation, where specific questions were asked regarding stroke changes and movement patterns causing symptoms to better understand the probable cause of the overuse injury. Placement of the patient in an evaluative situation, with a biomechanical or coaching authority who has demonstrated an expertise in the patient's sport, is therefore highly recommended.

Specifically, the interval tennis program is initiated through stroke simulation of the forehand and backhand with the racquet and no ball contact. Once the patient is able to tolerate this simulated stroke activity, ball impact is initiated using a foam "gator" ball (Wilson Sporting Goods Co., Elk Grove Village, IL). The rationale for using the foam ball is the lower impact stress, due to its lighter weight, imparted to the patient's extremity. Feeding the foam ball to the patient is recommended, with emphasis on a full stroke and proper form. The next stage in the program is actual groundstroke execution using a standard tennis ball. Balls are initially fed to the individual from the net to the baseline. Partner feeding ensures a more controlled and slower preimpact ball velocity, which minimizes impact stress to the injured area. Consistent with any interval return program, if the patient has symptoms or discomfort with any stage or level of the program, they are returned to a lower intensity, previously tolerated stage.

The general concept of the interval tennis program is a progression from lower levels of preimpact ball velocity and stress to more functional sport-specific stresses as the individual adapts to the activity. The patient attempts 20 to 30 repetitions of each stroke (forehand and backhand) and progresses in repetitions only after two to three successful exercise trials at each level. The next level in the interval tennis program includes rallying with a partner from baseline to baseline in a controlled fashion, again with emphasis on proper stroke mechanics and a full stroking pattern. A backboard is not used or recommended with the interval tennis program due to its fast and continual rebound characteristics, which encourage continued, uninterrupted muscle work in the upper extremity. Use of a ball machine is an acceptable substitute to rallying with a partner. Once several pain-free trials of rallying from the baseline are achieved, forehand and backhand volleys are initiated. As signs and symptoms allow, 15 to 20 volleys are mixed in among groundstrokes. Pain-free volleys and groundstrokes are prerequisites for progression to the serve and overhead.

A submaximal trial of serving is initiated, again with stroke simulation and foam ball impact. Initial velocity expectations are as low as 40 to 60 percent of normal volition to prevent injury. The overhead smash is added once the more controlled serving motion is tolerated by the patient. The number of repetitions and velocity are increased sequentially as muscular strength and endurance allow. The final step in the interval program is actual simulated match play. To progress to this step, the player's upper extremity should tolerate 1 hour of groundstroke and volley activity, as well as 40 to 50 serves during a workout.

Interval Throwing Return Program.   The interval throwing program developed by Wilk, Arrigo, and Andrews (1993) is presented in Appendix B, Interval Return Programs: Throwing. As with the interval tennis program, progressive increases in duration, intensity, and distance are controlled so that the stresses on the throwing elbow and upper extremity in general are increased sequentially. The 14-step program begins with easy tossing at 30 to 45 feet, again emphasizing proper mechanics with particular reference to whole-body contribution to the throwing motion and not merely "arming" the ball. The athlete's use of shoulder rotation as well as the "crow hop" (first a hop, then a skip, followed by a throw) method of delivery are monitored. Each stage progresses in the number of throwing repetitions and through gradual lengthening of the throwing distance as the intensity of the patient's effort is increased.

Participation in the interval throwing or tennis program is part of the rehabilitation process and is most often performed at the clinic to allow monitoring of the patient's mechanics and to ensure compliance with the throwing distance and intensity. Performance of the interval program at the clinic also allows for proper administration and assistance of the warm-up prior to throwing, as well as proper postworkout precautions, such as icing.

Wilk, Arrigo, and Andrews (1993) also have developed an additional progression for pitchers following completion of the initial 14-stage throwing program. A gradual progression is followed with the patient throwing only fastballs, initially at 50 to 75 percent of maximal effort and eventually at 100 percent of maximal velocity. Only then are breaking balls and simulated game activity introduced.

Successful application of the interval programs presented in this section relies on individual adaptation of the program to the patient. Significantly slower progressions of the interval programs are usually applied in postoperative rehabilitation or with rehabilitation of chronic tendon degenerative conditions, whereas a more rapid progression is followed in individuals with more advanced levels of muscle strength and neuromuscular coordination. The interval program developed by Wilk, Arrigo, and Andrews (1993) for prepubescent and adolescent age throwing athletes is contained in the "little leaguer" interval program (Appendix B, Interval Return Programs: Throwing).

Operative Treatment and Rehabilitation

In Nirschl's initial study of 3000 cases of humeral epicondylitis, 92 percent responded to nonoperative treatment. Characteristics seen in patients not responding to nonoperative treatment were chronic symptoms of pain, often in the contralateral shoulder and elbow; intense pain in the injured elbow, even at rest; tennis strokes requiring excessive forearm activity; short-term relief following cortisone injection; and exacerbation of symptoms with electrical stimulation (Nirschl & Sobel, 1981).

To better understand postoperative rehabilitation, a brief description of the surgery performed by Nirschl for humeral epicondylitis is presented.

Surgical Techniques

The incision used by Nirschl (1992) for lateral epicondylitis extends from the level of the radial head to 1 inch proximal to the lateral epicondyle (figure 6.14). Debridement of the angiofibroblastic degenerative tendinosis from the extensor brevis is commonly performed. All pathologic tissue is removed without disturbing the attachment of the extensor aponeurosis. A small opening is made in the lateral synovium to inspect the lateral compartment of the joint. Vascular enhancement is provided by drilling three

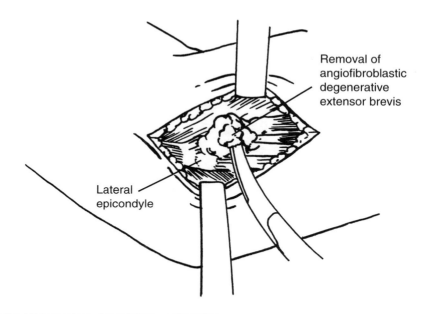

FIGURE 6.14 Lateral view of the elbow showing the removal of angiofibroblastic degeneration from the extensor carpi radialis brevis as described by Nirschl. Adapted from Morrey 1994.

holes through the cortical bone of the anterior lateral condyle to cancellous bone level.

The incision used by Nirschl for medial epicondylitis is approximately 3 inches in length and parallels the medial epicondylar groove. Again, resection of the angiofibroblastic tendinosis is performed, commonly localized to the pronator teres and flexor carpi radialis tendinous insertions (figure 6.15). The common flexor origin is not released, and due to its important function in stabilizing the medial aspect of the elbow, it remains intact.

In a prospective analysis of fifty cases of intractable medial epicondylitis, Ollivierre, Nirschl, and Pettrone (1995) identified angiofibroblastic tendinosis and fibrallary degeneration of collagen in the tendons of the flexor carpi radialis and pronator teres tendons. A follow-up averaging 37 months revealed that all fifty cases had partial or complete relief of symptoms, improved grip strength measured with a hand-held dynamometer, and no postoperative complications. The authors concluded that a large percentage of patients who fail conservative treatment can obtain both pain relief and return to functional activities with the operative technique described.

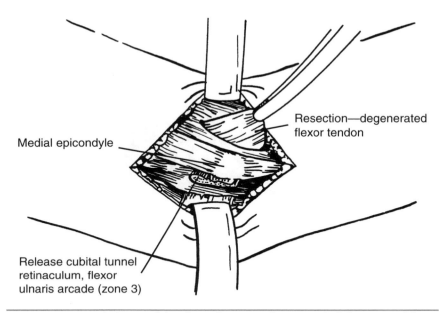

Resection—degenerated flexor tendon

Medial epicondyle

Release cubital tunnel retinaculum, flexor ulnaris arcade (zone 3)

FIGURE 6.15   Medial view of the elbow illustrating the removal of degenerated flexor tendon and release of the ulnar nerve as described by Nirschl. Adapted from Morrey 1994.

Nirschl reports that 60 percent of patients operated on for medial epicondylitis have symptoms reflective of ulnar nerve dysfunction. To address these symptoms, decompression of zone 3 (distal to the medial epicondyle) of the ulnar nerve is performed by release of the flexor carpi ulnaris arcade. Nirschl does not perform an ulnar nerve transposition unless valgus instability of the elbow is present, subluxation of the nerve from the epicondylar groove exists, excessive skeletal valgus is present, or further surgical exposure of the medial elbow necessitates transposition (Nirschl, 1992).

Several other operative techniques are presented in the literature. A modified Bosworth III is described and includes release of the extensor aponeurosis and the orbital ligament and excision of the bursae, if present, as well as the synovial fringe (Boyd & Mcleod, 1973). Stovall and Bernfield (1979) report good results performing an operation described by Garden consisting of lengthening of the extensor carpi radialis brevis just proximal to the wrist. Roles and Mawdsley (1972) reported on a series of 33 patients who responded to surgical decompression of the radial nerve. Impingement of the posterior interosseous nerve at the arcade of Frohse is a differential diagnosis for lateral epicondylitis and is thought to coexist with true lateral epicondylitis in about 5 percent of cases (Nirschl, 1992). Nirschl reports 85 percent excellent results, which include complete pain relief and full functional return in 750 cases of surgical treatment of humeral epicondylitis. In this group, 12 percent experience significant pain relief and a return to vigorous sports, but not complete normalcy. Three percent had no change in symptoms or improvement in strength.

Postoperative Rehabilitation

The primary stages of rehabilitation previously discussed for humeral epicondylitis are used in the postoperative rehabilitation of lateral, medial, and posterior tennis elbow (see pages 90-116). The protocol for postoperative rehabilitation recommended by Nirschl is presented in Appendix A, Postoperative Protocols: Humeral Epicondylitis.

Postoperatively, the patient is placed in an immobilizer in 90° of elbow flexion at all times for seven days, with occasional use of the immobilizer for protection for the first three weeks thereafter. Limbering exercises for the wrist and fingers are initiated on day 2. On days 3 through 6, gentle motion of the elbow is performed. Elbow range of motion is progressed gradually such that by day 17, 80 percent of full range is achieved.

Approximately three weeks after surgery, resistive exercise is initiated using isometrics and manual resistance, as well as activities such as squeezing a Nerf ball. Light weights are added, along with isotonic exercise patterns identical to those used in nonoperative rehabilitation. A counterforce brace is used during performance of the exercises and activities of daily living. Return of full dominant arm strength after surgery averages four and a half months for lateral epicondylitis and posterior tennis elbow and five and a half months for medial epicondylitis (Nirschl, 1992). Interval sport return programs are started as early as six weeks after surgery, but a full return of strength is recommended before competitive racquet sport and throwing activity commences.

Osteochondral Injury (Removal of Loose Bodies/Debridement)

Treatment of the elbow with significant osteochondral injury often begins with nonoperative measures to control pain and inflammation as well as to maintain or improve joint arthrokinematics. Modification of the individual's activity often temporarily relieves symptoms; however, the true underlying cause of the osteochondral injury, such as ulnohumeral joint instability, osseous spur development, and abnormal sport or ADL mechanical stresses, makes nonoperative rehabilitation a less effective total treatment choice for this classification of injury. As with other musculoskeletal injuries in the athletic elbow, nonoperative rehabilitation is often attempted and, although unsuccessful with respect to resolution of symptoms, prepares the elbow for surgical treatment options by increasing strength and range of motion and decreasing pain preoperatively.

Elbow Arthroscopy

Elbow arthroscopy is indicated for many surgical procedures about the elbow. One of the most common arthroscopic procedures in the athletic elbow is the removal of lesions of the posterior compartment, specifically loose bodies (Andrews, 1985; Andrews & Craven, 1991). Loose bodies can be floating freely about the joint or held in place by reactive synovitis. The pathomechanics that result in formation of these loose bodies are valgus extension overload forces and additional stress on the tip of the olecranon imparted by the violently contracting triceps tendon during the throwing or serving motion. The combined valgus extension force pattern can cause formation of these posterior bony lesions, and the body's reaction to the stresses (Wolff's law) can contribute to additional lesions as well (Andrews & Craven, 1991). Table 6.1 lists the most common elbow arthroscopy diagnoses seen in a population of 467 patients (Timmerman & Andrews, 1994a).

Arthroscopy has been the single most important surgical advance in the aggressive treatment of athletic injuries requiring surgical intervention. Arthroscopic procedures for the elbow have, without doubt, greatly accelerated the return to sport activity and prolonged individual athletic careers. Elbow arthroscopy permits improved visualization of the joint's intra-articular pathology while decreasing the amount of dissection, tissue disruption, and morbidity. This combination has allowed for both improved diagnostic abilities and a quicker return to aggressive rehabilitation. Elbow arthroscopy, however, is technically demanding for the orthopedic

TABLE 6.1   Elbow Arthroscopy Diagnoses in 467 Patients (1980-1992)

Postoperative diagnosis	Number of patients
Osteophytes	218
Loose bodies	181
Valgus extension overload	131
Medial (ulnar) collateral ligament strain or tear	70
Osteochondritis dissecans	38
Synovitis	31
Posttraumatic arthrofibrosis	30
Degenerative joint disease	18
Other	58

Reprinted from Andrews and Soffer 1994.

surgeon, and the potential for surgical complications is great. Elbow arthroscopy requires in-depth knowledge of elbow anatomy, well-trained surgical skills, and the best of surgical judgment.

A more complete description of elbow arthroscopy is given in the next section to enhance the understanding of clinicians regarding portal placement, possible complications of portal sites, and postoperative rehabilitative emphases based on this procedure.

Surgical Techniques

Arthroscopy of the elbow can be performed with the patient in the supine or prone position. If the supine position is employed, a traction suspension device is used to suspend and position the elbow for arthroscopy. The surgeon should first palpate and mark with a pen the bony landmarks about the elbow. This ensures appropriate placement of arthroscopic portals (incisions) and helps avoid vital structures.

Direct lateral and anterolateral portals.   The joint is initially distended with sterile fluid with a needle inserted into the direct lateral portal, a "soft point" central to a triangle formed by the radial head, lateral epicondyle, and olecranon tip (figure 6.16). No major neurovascular structures normally occupy this triangle. The joint is initially entered through the anterolateral portal, which is located 2-3 cm distal to and 1 cm anterior to the lateral epicondyle and anterior to the radial head (Andrews, St. Pierre, & Carson, 1986) (figure 6.17a). This point should be palpated while ranging the radial capitellar joint in supination and pronation. At this point, the arthroscopic portal penetrates the extensor wad and extensor carpi radialis near the radial nerve (figure 6.17b). The radial nerve is approximately 4 mm from this portal without joint distention and approximately 11 mm with the joint distended with fluid (Lynch, Meyers, Whipple, & Caspari, 1986). The posterior antebrachial cutaneous nerve lies approximately 2 mm from this area.

Anteromedial portal.   The anteromedial portal has been described by Andrews & McKenzie (1991) at a point 2 cm anterior and 2 cm distal to the medial epicondyle (figure 6.18a). The flexor muscle mass is entered between the flexor digitorum superficialis and flexor carpi radialis, then through the pronator teres and into the elbow joint (figure 6.18b). Flexion of the elbow allows for further avoidance of the median nerve and median and brachial arteries (Lynch et al., 1986).

Posterolateral portal.   The posterolateral portal is usually the initial entry point into the posterior compartment of the elbow. The elbow is extended to help relax the triceps tendon. The point of entry is 3 cm proximal to the olecranon tip and just lateral to the lateral edge of the triceps (figure 6.19). The path is through the triceps muscle toward the olecranon fossa. It

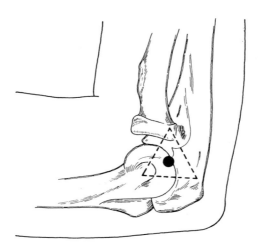

FIGURE 6.16   Direct lateral arthroscopic portal location bordered by the lateral humeral epicondyle, radial head, and tip of the olecranon. Reprinted from Andrews and Soffer 1994.

should be remembered that the ulnar nerve is medial to the medial aspect of the triceps muscle.

Posterior portal.   Andrews describes using a direct posterior working portal located approximately 3 cm proximal to the olecranon tip, penetrating the triceps tendon (figure 6.19). This portal allows surgical procedures in the posterior compartment, such as removing loose bodies from the posterior aspect of the elbow or resection of an impinging olecranon osteophyte (figure 6.20).

Rehabilitation Following Elbow Arthroscopy

Patients are often placed in a sling postoperatively for approximately 24 to 48 hours. An injection of local anesthetic normally given to the joint following arthroscopy of the knee and shoulder is not generally administered because of the potential for radial or median peripheral nerve block with fluid extravasation (Chase & Baker, 1994).

Gentle movements of the elbow, forearm, wrist, and fingers are allowed, with physical therapy often commencing on the first or second postoperative day. Passive and active-assisted range of motion are started with gentle grade I or II mobilizations to assist in both range-of-motion attainment and pain management. Range of motion to terminal ranges can be performed if tolerated in the elbow, forearm, and wrist. Shoulder range of

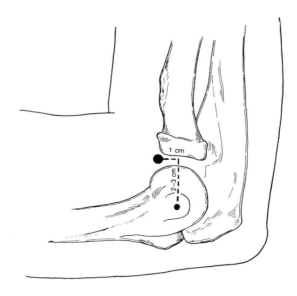

a

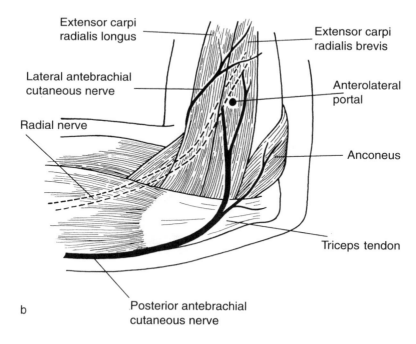

Extensor carpi
radialis longus

Extensor carpi
radialis brevis

Lateral antebrachial
cutaneous nerve

Anterolateral
portal

Radial nerve

Anconeus

Triceps tendon

b

Posterior antebrachial
cutaneous nerve

FIGURE 6.17   Location and surrounding structure of the anterolateral arthroscopic portal site showing proximity to the joint (a) and to the radial nerve (b). Reprinted from Andrews and Soffer 1994.

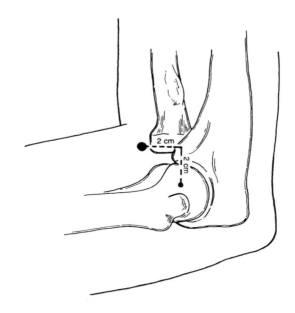

a

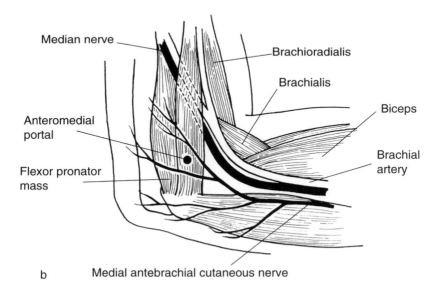

Median nerve

Brachioradialis

Brachialis

Biceps

Anteromedial portal

Brachial artery

Flexor pronator mass

b   Medial antebrachial cutaneous nerve

FIGURE 6.18   Anteromedial arthroscopic portal site showing proximity to the medial epicondyle (a) and the related anatomical structures (b). Reprinted from Andrews and Soffer 1994.

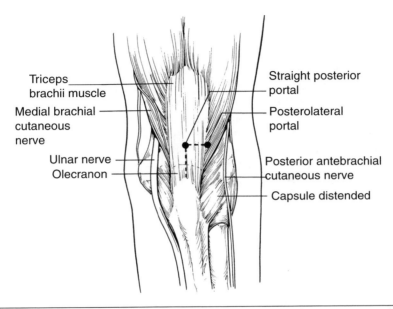

FIGURE 6.19   Location of posterolateral and posterior arthroscopic portals. Reprinted from Esch and Baker 1993.

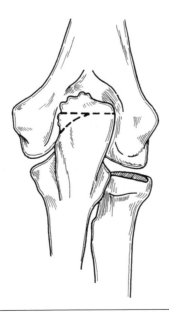

FIGURE 6.20   Posterior view of the elbow with dotted line depicting resection of the posterior olecranon tip. Reprinted from Andrews and Soffer 1994.

motion should also be addressed to prevent contracture and the negative effects of disuse. Grip putty is used for gross wrist and hand strengthening and is prescribed for home exercise.

By the third postoperative day, full range of motion is often achieved and light resistive exercise can be initiated. The patterns used with nonoperative rehabilitation of humeral epicondylitis are also employed using no weight or as little as 1 to 2 pounds. Again, a low- or no-resistance, high-repetition (30 to 45 reps per exercise) format is used to minimize the chance of increasing pain, yet beginning the neuromuscular exchange inherent in resistive exercise. Initial resistive exercises of the forearm and wrist are performed in a comfortable, midrange position with the elbow in approximately 70° of flexion. Elbow extension/flexion resistive exercises are not performed into full extension for the first two to three weeks postoperatively, especially after debridement of the posterior compartment. The progression of resistive exercise continues through the first four weeks following surgery with the total arm strength concept, including glenohumeral and scapulothoracic exercise patterns.

Initiation of isokinetic exercise is warranted at four weeks after surgery using the progression from wrist flexion/extension to forearm pronation/supination. Controlled isotonic exercise in the distal patterns discussed previously, with a 5-pound dumbbell or medium-level rubber tubing, as well as full, pain-free range of available motion are required prior to isokinetic introduction. Plyometric and closed-chain exercise sequences are also used as outlined for humeral epicondylitis. Progression to an interval throwing or tennis program begins between four and eight weeks after surgery. See the protocol for postoperative rehabilitation following elbow arthroscopy in Appendix A, Postoperative Protocols: Arthroscopic Debridement/Removal of Loose Bodies.

Clinical Outcome Studies: Elbow Arthroscopy

In a follow-up study of 71 cases of elbow arthroscopy, O'Driscoll and Morrey (1992) reported success in 75 percent of patients with loose bodies and an 80 percent success rate for joint debridement. The early use of range of motion and rapid progression of resistive exercise following the less invasive arthroscopic approach to elbow surgery assists both the patient and clinician during rehabilitation. Ogilvie-Harris, Gordon, and MacKay (1995) reported excellent results in 14 of 21 patients who underwent arthroscopic treatment for posterior impingement associated with degenerative arthritis and good results in the remaining seven patients. The arthroscopic procedure consisted of three parts: removal of posterior loose bodies, removal of posterior olecranon osteophytes, and removal of osteophytes in the olecranon fossa to the point of fenestration. Patients had an average follow-up of 35 months and were graded using Morrey's 100-Point Classification System (see Appendix C), which uses pain, motion, strength, instability, and function as primary factors in postoperative or postinjury outcome (Morrey, Askew, An, & Chao, 1981). The authors concluded that arthroscopic treatment for posterior impingement in the degenerative elbow provides substantial improvement with minimal risk.

Andrews and Timmerman (1995) reviewed the records of 72 professional baseball players who underwent either arthroscopic or open elbow surgery on their throwing arm. The most common diagnoses reviewed were posteromedial osteophytes (65 percent) and ulnar collateral ligament injury (25 percent). Eighty percent of the players were able to return to play for a minimum of one season following surgery; 25 percent of the players required two or more surgical procedures, with 25 percent of those procedures being ulnar collateral ligament reconstruction. The high incidence of reoperation on the patients who initially underwent arthroscopic posteromedial osteophyte debridement demonstrates the close association between laxity in the medial collateral ligament and osseous pathology on the posterior medial olecranon and trochlea. Andrews and Timmerman (1995) conclude that the initial incidence of ulnar collateral ligament injury was underestimated.

Ulnar Nerve Dysfunction (Neuritis)

The biomechanical stresses imparted to the medial aspect of the elbow with repetitive overhead activities can lead to inflammation and mechanical irritation of the ulnar nerve at the elbow (Joyce et al., 1995). Ligamentous instability, as well as insufficient anatomical stabilization of the ulnar nerve leading to subluxation, can potentially increase the athlete's susceptibility to ulnar nerve injury. Initial nonoperative rehabilitation of the patient with ulnar neuritis is indicated, with ulnar nerve transposition being used in refractory cases.

Nonoperative Treatment and Rehabilitation

The nonoperative treatment stages and exercise progression for the athlete with ulnar neuritis parallel those for humeral epicondylitis (see pages 90-116). Great care must be taken during the initial evaluation to rule out the presence of ligamentous instability or obvious skeletal valgus, which compromise the neural structures on the medial aspect of the elbow. Hypermobility and subluxation or dislocation of the ulnar nerve must also be tested to further delineate the source of ulnar nerve irritation. Particular attention is paid to the distal distribution of the ulnar nerve at the

SURGICAL APPROACHES TO THE ELBOW

Basic knowledge of the common surgical approaches to the elbow enhances the understanding of the rehabilitative protocols and specific structures that need emphasis following an open surgical procedure.

Lateral Approach

Prior to the evolution of elbow arthroscopy, this approach was commonly used for the removal of loose bodies through an arthrotomy. It is still employed for this purpose when necessary. A curved incision is made over the lateral epicondyle. An interval is developed between the anconeus and extensor carpi ulnaris distally and the lateral edge of the triceps tendon proximally. Dissection of the anconeus subposteriorally, followed by its release from the triceps, exposes the joint's lateral ligamentous structures. With range of motion of the elbow into extension, the tip of the olecranon can be approached for possible osteophyte resection. Loose bodies are commonly found in this posterior compartment.

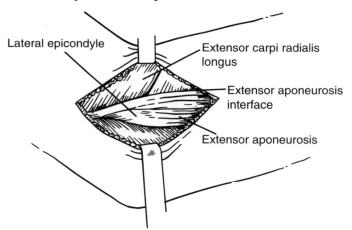

Figure 6.5.1 Lateral view of the elbow showing the lateral skin incision and further dissection of the lateral open surgical approach. From Morrey 1994.

Anterior Approach

Henry (1957) described the open anterior surgical approach to the elbow. Repair of distally ruptured biceps tendons employs this approach, which is made between the biceps and brachialis medially and brachioradialis laterally. There is an interval distally between the pronator teres and the brachioradialis. The radial nerve found along the inner surface of the brachioradialis should be identified and protected.

Posterior Approach

A triceps-splitting approach just lateral to the tip of the olecranon is used to approach the posterior olecranon osteophytes and triceps tendon calcific deposits. It is crucial to avoid the ulnar nerve medially and the radial nerve, which lies approximately 8 cm above or proximal to the lateral epicondyle.

Medial Approach

Approach to the medial aspect of the elbow is usually centered around the medial epicondyle. A curvilinear incision centered over the medial epicondyle can allow ulnar nerve decompression and transposition, repair of fractures, surgery for chronic inflammation, and medial ulnar collateral ligament repair or reconstruction.

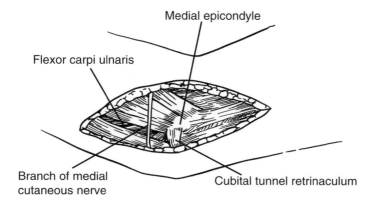

Figure 6.5.2   Medial view of the elbow demonstrating the medial open surgical approach to the elbow. From Morrey 1994.

During the medial approach, the medial antebrachial cutaneous nerve is protected in an attempt to prevent possible neuroma formation. The ulnar nerve is then identified for protection or eventual decompression or transposition. The medial ulnar collateral ligament can be exposed through a splitting incision by detaching the musculotendinous insertion of the flexor/pronator group on the medial epicondyle.

hypothenar eminence of the hand, continuing into the fifth finger and ulnar side of the fourth digit. Changes in sensation and subjective reports of pain or paresthesia in these distal regions, in addition to the local symptoms at the ulnar groove, govern the progression or regression of physical therapy, including resistive exercise. Repeated reassessment of the motor and sensory distributions of the ulnar nerve's distal course must be performed via light touch sensation and manual muscle testing.

Use of modalities to decrease pain and inflammation is warranted in the local region of the ulnar nerve at the elbow. Mobilization and passive stretching are also performed to normalize length tension relationships of the flexor/pronator musculature and promote the reattainment of elbow extension (the position of osseous congruency and stability). Low-resistance, high-repetition exercises are employed as signs and symptoms allow, employing distal strengthening patterns similar to those used for humeral epicondylitis. Total arm strength exercises are also used for the scapulothoracic and scapulohumeral musculature, with resistance applied in a manner that does not either produce undue valgus stress or attenuate the ulnar nerve. Isokinetic exercise and interval functional return programs are also used in the later stages of rehabilitation.

Continued ulnar nerve instability, distal neural symptoms, and pain that limits performance despite a comprehensive nonoperative rehabilitation program make the patient a candidate for surgical transposition or decompression of the ulnar nerve.

Operative Treatment

To relieve discomfort of the chronically inflamed or subluxing ulnar nerve in the athletic elbow, the ulnar nerve can be decompressed and or transposed anteriorly. We prefer subcutaneous positioning of the ulnar nerve in created fascial slings, although the nerve can be transposed submuscularly.

Through the medial surgical procedure (see page 129), the ulnar nerve is mobilized after incising the fascia of the cubital tunnel. Care is taken to decompress and mobilize the ulnar nerve proximally to the level of the arcade of Struthers. Distally, the intermuscular septum is excised to allow anterior transposition. Motor branches should be carefully protected and preserved. Fascial slings are created from the fascia overlying the tendinous insertion of the flexor/pronator muscle group on the medial epicondyle (figure 6.21). The transposed ulnar nerve is placed loosely under these fascial slings, avoiding acute angulation and impingement, even during directly observed range of motion during surgery. The 25- to 30-mm by 6- to 12-mm fascial slings are created, leaving them patent on the medial epicondyle. The underlying muscle tissue is dissected, freeing the fascial layer. The fascial defects are repaired to prevent herniation, and the distal aspects of the flaps are reattached loosely over the transposed ulnar nerve. For optimal results, it is crucial to decompress the ulnar nerve adequately, both proximally and distally. A well-padded compression dressing with posterior splinting of the elbow at neutral 90° positioning is recommended intraoperatively.

Rettig and Ebben (1993) reported on 21 cases of ulnar nerve transposition in athletes. The average time for return to full activity was 12.6 weeks postsurgery. Full range of motion and normal two-point discrimination were present in 100 percent of the cases at the six-week postoperative examination. The authors conclude that the use of an ulnar nerve transposition using fascial slings is a successful and safe method for treating patients with ulnar neuritis as well as ulnar nerve subluxation.

Postoperative Rehabilitation

The postoperative protocol following ulnar nerve transposition is listed in Appendix A, Postoperative Protocols: Ulnar Nerve Transposition. The patient is immobilized in a posterior splint or hinged elbow brace to allow

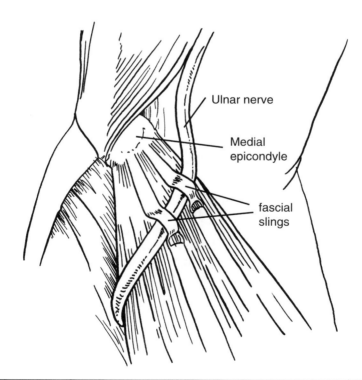

Ulnar nerve

Medial epicondyle

fascial slings

FIGURE 6.21   Medial view of the elbow showing fascial slings used to transpose the ulnar nerve.

the soft tissues to heal and to provide limited motion about the elbow in a safe, neutral range of motion. During the first postoperative week, the patient's brace is set from -30° of extension to 100° of elbow flexion. Selective distal range of motion is performed into forearm pronation and wrist flexion, with guarded wrist extension and forearm supination to protect the flexor/pronator origin. Gentle isometrics with extremely light resistance levels are applied to prevent disuse atrophy. Foam ball or putty squeezing is also used.

During week 2, range of motion is progressed to -15° of elbow extension and 120° of elbow flexion. Gentle manual resistance and distal strengthening patterns, using little or no weight, are applied as tolerated. During week 3, the immobilizer is opened to allow full range of motion with continued use of light isotonic strengthening using patterns identical to those presented for the nonoperative rehabilitation of humeral epicondylitis (see pages 90-116). Range of motion of the glenohumeral joint continues throughout rehabilitation to prevent contractures from disuse. During week 6, isotonic shoulder and scapular strengthening exercises are begun, with resistance being applied proximal to the elbow to prevent excessive stress across the elbow.

Isokinetic wrist and forearm exercise is initiated at 10 weeks postoperatively, with progression to interval sport return programs by week 12. An isokinetic evaluation is performed at this time to formally assess strength of the wrist and forearm musculature. A shoulder isokinetic test is also performed to assess more proximally the relative strength and balance of strength prior to performing interval sport return programs.

Ulnar Collateral Ligament Injury

Injury to the ulnar collateral ligament from the repetitive valgus stresses inherent in upper extremity sport activity results in either nonoperative or operative management. In the patient with a mild sprain of the ulnar collateral ligament, nonoperative rehabilitation serves to decrease pain and inflammation as well as restore necessary range of motion and strength. Patients not responding to nonoperative treatment and those with excessive valgus instability of the elbow are most successfully treated with ulnar collateral ligament reconstruction and extensive postoperative rehabilitation.

Nonoperative Rehabilitation

Attenuation of the ulnar collateral ligament can produce valgus instability of the elbow, which can lead to medial joint pain, ulnar nerve compromise, and lateral radiocapitellar and posterolateral osseous dysfunction, which is a severely restricting injury to the throwing or racquet sport athlete.

Nonoperative rehabilitation of the athlete with an ulnar collateral ligament sprain also involves the primary stage outlined for rehabilitation of humeral epicondylitis (see pages 90-94). During the initial stage of rehabilitation, the elbow is often immobilized to decrease pain and enhance healing. Either an immobilizer or a hinged brace is used to limit end ranges of elbow extension and flexion. Modalities are again used to assist in the healing process, as is gentle range-of-motion and submaximal isometric and manual resistance of both wrist and forearm midrange movements.

A total arm strength rehabilitation protocol is also indicated to facilitate both muscular strength and endurance in the elbow, forearm, and wrist (see pages 94-114). In addition to previously mentioned exercises, particular attention is paid to eccentric muscle work of the wrist flexors and forearm supinators so as to dynamically support the attenuated ulnar collateral ligament. Due to the intimate association between the flexor carpi ulnaris and the ulnar collateral ligament, early strengthening in the pattern of wrist flexion and ulnar deviation may provoke symptoms; however, later in rehabilitation, the repeated use of exercises to strengthen the muscles directly overlying the injured ligament is highly recommended to provide dynamic stabilization (Davidson et al., 1995).

Progression to plyometric exercises that impart a submaximal, controlled valgus stress to the medial aspect of the elbow, such as a 90/90 shoulder and elbow medicine ball toss, in later stages of rehabilitation attempt to simulate loads placed on the medial elbow (see figures 6.9 and 6.10). Use of the isokinetic dynamometer for distal strengthening is also recommended, with additional training focused on the shoulder for internal/external rotation with the arm abducted 90° and the elbow flexed 90° (figure 6.22). This position imparts a controlled valgus stress to the elbow, in addition to strengthening the rotator cuff (Ellenbecker, Davies, & Rowinski, 1988).

A complete return of range of motion and isokinetically documented elbow, forearm, and wrist strength is required before an interval program is initiated. Reoccurrence of pain, feelings of instability, or neural irritation with throwing or functional activity identify the patient as a potential candidate for ulnar collateral ligament repair or reconstruction.

Operative Management

Operative procedures for the athlete with valgus instability of the elbow have focused on direct primary repair of the ligament (Kuroda & Sakamaki, 1986) as well as on use of an autogenous graft for reconstruction of the medial elbow (Conway et al., 1992; Jobe, Stark, & Lombardo, 1986). Regan, Korinek, Morrey, and An (1991) reported that the palmaris tendon used as the autogenous graft, harvested from the ipsilateral forearm, fails at higher

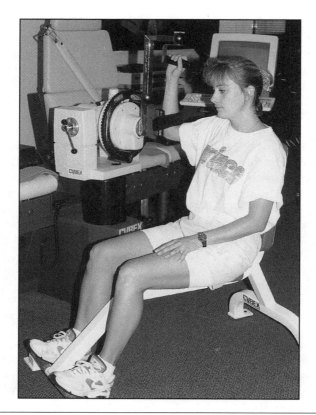

FIGURE 6.22 Isokinetic training movement pattern for internal and external rotation with the shoulder in 90° of abduction in the scapular plane. Use of this pattern exposes the medial aspect of the elbow to a controlled valgus stress.

loads (357 N) and is four times as strong as the anterior band of the ulnar collateral ligament, which fails at 260 N.

In a retrospective study by Conway et al. (1992) of 71 throwing athletes who underwent either surgical repair or reconstruction of the ulnar collateral ligament, 87 percent were found to have a midsubstance tear of the ulnar collateral ligament, 10 percent had a distal ulnar avulsion, and only 3 percent avulsed from the medial epicondyle. Of these athletic elbows, 39 percent had calcification and scar formation in the ulnar collateral ligament, with 16 percent demonstrating an osteophyte to the posteromedial olecranon, most likely due to the increased valgus extension overload secondary to ulnar collateral ligament attenuation.

Preoperative clinical evaluation of these patients resulted in a positive valgus stress test in 8 of 14 patients who underwent ulnar collateral ligament repair and 33 of 56 patients who underwent autogenous reconstruction. Valgus stress radiographs were also used in the preoperative evaluation, with greater emphasis placed on the subjective and clinical evaluation (Conway et al., 1992). Fifty percent of these athletes demonstrated a flexion contracture that limited full elbow extension.

Surgical Techniques

The surgical technique used to reconstruct the ulnar collateral ligament is described extensively by Conway et al. (1992), Jobe and Elattrache (1993), and Jobe, Stark, and Lombardo (1986). A 10-cm medial incision is made over the medial epicondyle to provide exposure, with careful dissection and protection of the ulnar nerve carried out before the ulnar collateral ligament is addressed. If a primary repair is performed, adequate normal-appearing ligamentous tissue is required to allow for direct repair. If inadequate ligamentous tissue is present, a reconstruction is performed. Additional exposure is required to perform the reconstruction, which is obtained by transection of the flexor/pronator tendinous origin.

This has important ramifications with respect to rehabilitation. Removal of this tendinous origin results in more time being required for healing and a lengthier period before resistive exercise of the flexor/pronator muscles and forearm supination and wrist extension range of motion can be performed.

Calcification within the ligament and surrounding soft tissues is also removed, with relocation of the ulnar nerve performed by removing it from the cubital tunnel. The ulnar nerve is mobilized from the level of the arcade of Struthers to the interval between the two heads of the flexor carpi ulnaris. The attachment sites of the anterior band of the ulnar collateral ligament are identified, and tunnels are drilled in the medial epicondyle and proximal ulna to approximate the anatomical location of the original ligament. The graft taken from the ipsilateral palmaris longus (if available) is then placed in a figure-of-eight fashion through the tunnels (figure 6.23). The ulnar nerve is carefully transposed so that no impingement or tethering occurs. The flexor/pronator origin is then reattached. The elbow is immobilized in a position of 90° of flexion and neutral forearm rotation, with the wrist left free to move.

Postoperative Rehabilitation

Following reconstruction of the ulnar collateral ligament using autogenous graft, the elbow remains immobilized for the first 10 days, with gentle gripping exercises allowed to prevent further disuse atrophy. Active and passive range of motion of the elbow, wrist, and shoulder are performed at 10 days following surgery. Close monitoring of the ulnar nerve distribution in the distal upper extremity is recommended due to the recent transposition of

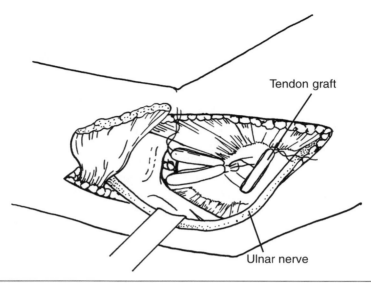

Tendon graft

Ulnar nerve

FIGURE 6.23   Medial view of the elbow showing reconstruction of the ulnar collateral ligament with autogenous graft. A figure-of-eight orientation is used to reconstruct the medial elbow. Adapted from Jobe and Elattrache 1993.

the nerve. Appendix A, Postoperative Protocols: Ulnar Collateral Ligament Reconstruction Using Autogenous Graft, lists examples of postoperative protocols following such reconstruction (Seto, Brewster, Randall, & Jobe, 1991; Wilk, Arrigo, & Andrews, 1993; Wilk, Azar, & Andrews, 1995).

As discussed in the surgical summary above, care is taken to protect the graft by gradually progressing elbow extension range of motion to 30° by week 2 and finally to terminal ranges by four to six weeks after surgery. Protection of the graft from large stresses is recommended, even though loss of extension range of motion is an undesirable postoperative result. Therefore, progressive increases in elbow extension range of motion and the use of gentle joint mobilization and contract-relax stretching techniques are warranted to achieve timely, optimal elbow extension (see pages 66-68). Due to the reattachment of the flexor/pronator tendinous insertion, limited range of motion into wrist extension and forearm supination is performed for the first six weeks until healing of the flexor-pronator insertion takes place.

Rehabilitation of the postoperative elbow should also include activities to restore proprioceptive function to the injured joint. Kinesthesia is the perceived sensation of the position and movement of joints and muscles and is important in the coordination of movement patterns in the peripheral joints. Simple exercises such as angular replication and end-range reproduction can be used early in rehabilitation, without visual assistance, to stimulate mechanoreceptors in the postoperative joint. These procedures are used early in the rehabilitation process concomitant with range of motion and joint mobilization. Loss of kinesthetic awareness in the upper extremity following injury has been identified objectively by Smith & Brunolli (1989).

The progression of resistive exercise follows previously discussed patterns (see pages 95-108), beginning with multiple-angle isometrics at week 2 and submaximal isotonics during the fourth postoperative week. Use of the total arm strength concept is followed, with proximal weight attachment for glenohumeral exercises to prevent stresses placed across the elbow. No glenohumeral joint internal or external rotation strengthening is allowed for at least 6 weeks to as many as 16 weeks after surgery due to the valgus stress placed on the elbow with this movement pattern. From 8 to 12 weeks following surgery, both concentric and eccentric exercises are performed in the elbow extensors and flexors, and there is continued emphasis on total arm strengthening, with all distal movement patterns described in nonoperative rehabilitation of humeral epicondylitis being applied (see pages 90-116). Plyometric exercises, ball dribbling, and closed-chain exercises are also used during this time frame.

Isokinetic training is introduced at four months after surgery, with isokinetic testing applied to identify areas needing specific emphasis (Wilk, Arrigo, & Andrews, 1993; Wilk et al., 1995). The progression of isokinetic training patterns we use again follows from wrist extension/flexion to forearm pronation/supination and, finally, elbow extension/flexion. The isokinetic dynamometer is also used at four to six months postoperatively for shoulder internal/external rotation strengthening with 90° of abduction and 90° of elbow flexion to impart a gentle, controlled valgus stress to the elbow. At four months after surgery, throwing athletes begin an interval throwing program to prepare the elbow for the stresses of functional activity. Specifics regarding the progression of the interval throwing program and progression to pitching are included in the protocols discussed earlier (see Appendix A, Postoperative Protocols: Ulnar Nerve Transposition, and Appendix B, Interval Return Programs: Throwing).

The postoperative duration of rehabilitation is often six months to a year. A slow revascularization of the graft through a sheath of granulation tissue that grows from the tissue adjacent to the site of implantation and encircles the graft is the rationale provided by Jobe, Stark, and Lombardo (1986) for their time-based rehabilitation program. They are convinced that at least one year is required for the tendon graft and its surrounding tissues to develop sufficient strength and endurance to function as a ligament in the medial elbow.

Clinical Outcomes

In their series of 56 reconstructed elbows, Conway et al. (1992) reported that baseball players return to throwing 15 feet by four and a half months, with competition at 12.5 months after surgery. The athlete with a repaired ulnar collateral ligament performed throwing activities of 15 feet at three months and competed at nine months. Overall, an excellent result was achieved in 64 percent of the elbows operated on (achieving a level of activity equal to or greater than preinjury) in elite athletes by Conway et al. (1992). Bennett, Green, and Tullos (1992) reported improved stability in 13 of 14 cases of ulnar collateral ligament reconstruction in an active adult working population, with improved stability reported in all cases of direct repair by Kuroda and Sakamaki (1986). Conway et al. (1992) reported a flexion contracture in as many as 50 percent of the athletes at a mean of six years following an autogenous ulnar collateral ligament reconstruction. They did not feel that this finding limits performance, because elbow range of motion during throwing ranges from 120° to 20°, although conscious effort is given to regaining as much extension as possible during the time-based rehabilitation program.

The use of extensive, endurance-oriented muscular strengthening exercises for the entire upper extremity is clearly warranted following elbow surgery. King et al. (1969) reported that valgus stresses to the elbow are first transmitted to the surrounding musculature and then to the medial ligaments of the elbow itself. The important role of the flexor/pronator muscle group in dynamically supporting the medial elbow is the primary rationale for inclusion of this extensive, exercise-oriented approach to elbow rehabilitation. It is important to reiterate the results of Glousman et al. (1992), which did not show increased EMG activity of the flexor/pronator muscles in the elbows of athletes with ulnar collateral ligament pathology. Once the ligament is injured, the dynamic stabilization provided by the medial musculature may be decreased through neural inhibition or other factors. Therefore, a complete approach to the unstable elbow, often including surgery and a thorough rehabilitation program, may be required to return elite levels of function to the elbow of the upper extremity sport athlete.

Growth Plate Injury

The stresses imparted to the adolescent throwing elbow can cause overuse injury to the epiphyseal plates. Treatment of growth plate injuries due to overuse, including nondisplaced fractures, is nonoperative (Joyce et al., 1995). Protection of the elbow from the stresses of throwing, limited immobilization, and modality application are all part of the initial treatment program. Progression of the patient to a total arm strength upper extremity program of resistive exercise follows the initial decrease of pain and inflammation required to promote healing and return the athlete to throwing. Evaluation of the adolescent athlete's mechanics is an integral part of the treatment program, with the regulation of both pitch count and frequency of aggressive throwing or overhead activity essential for preventing recurrence.

Operative Treatment and Rehabilitation

Rather than rupturing the medial ulnar collateral ligamentous complex, the skeletally immature athlete often avulses the medial epicondyle at its physis. Operative treatment is recommended for displaced fracture of the medial epicondyle using open reduction internal fixation (ORIF).

A standard medial approach allows pinning or preferably screw fixation of this injury. The ulnar nerve is usually protected and left patent. A posterior splint is used for approximately one week postoperatively, with rehabilitation initially focusing on retarding muscle atrophy of the distal muscle groups during immobilization and passive range of motion of joints proximal and distal to the elbow. Progression of range of motion and strengthening of the elbow following this procedure is similar to rehabilitation of the elbow following ulnar collateral ligament repair (see pages 135-138). Movement patterns and exercises that create a valgus stress on the elbow are avoided until complete healing of the fracture site is achieved (see Case Presentation 5, pages 156-159).

Case Presentations

As a final reinforcement of the total arm strength rehabilitation principles discussed in this book, we present case studies of patients who underwent five common rehabilitation courses following an overuse injury to the dominant elbow. Use of the total arm strength program and progression of resistance exercise in preparation for an interval return to activity are evident. The presentation of these cases highlights the objective clinical findings regarding range of motion and strength, important in every rehabilitative effort.

Lateral Epicondylitis

Subjective History

The patient is a 28-year-old right-handed female competitive tennis player and United States Professional Tennis Association certified teaching pro who presents with a two-week history of localized pain in the lateral aspect of the right elbow. Patient reports the pain to be localized to the lateral epicondyle and occasionally into the extensor surface of the forearm. The pain is rated a 5/10 at rest, and 8/10 with tennis play, teaching, or heavy forearm use such as typing or housework. The primary tennis strokes which create the patient's symptoms are the backhand groundstroke and backhand volley. She has minimal pain with forehands or serving. She denies any one incident of injury but reports playing competitive tournaments for her ranking the last three weeks in a row, as well as maintaining a heavy tennis teaching schedule at her club. She recently (2 months ago) changed tennis racquets, to a stiffer mid-sized frame. She reports that she strings her racquet at 65 pounds with synthetic gut string which is within the manufacturer's recommended tension range. She has tried icing and heating her elbow with little progress. She denies any neural radiation of symptoms and reports that she is taking an anti-inflammatory medication prescribed by her physician. X-rays taken during her physician visit were negative for osseous deformity. The patient has been playing tennis for 20 years, and does not report any recent change in her stroke mechanics. She feels as if her elbow is more sore during teaching which she does at times for 6-8 hours without breaks. The patient reports no previous upper extremity injury history or medical history.

Initial Exam Findings

The patient shows no visible atrophy in the right forearm and no visible swelling or ecchymosis. There is distinct, localized tenderness to palpation of the lateral epicondyle, and approximately 1-2 inches distal onto the extensor mass of the forearm. Negative varus and valgus stress tests are present bilaterally, negative good-hands test, negative Tinel's test, and a negative radiocapitellar compression test bilaterally. A positive extensor provocation test is present on the right elbow, with replication of the patient's symptoms. Negative flexor provocation is present bilaterally. Gross manual muscle testing shows 5/5 strength of elbow flexors and extensors, wrist flexors, and forearm pronators and supinators, 5-/5 strength in the wrist and finger extensors, particularly when tested with the elbow near full extension. Manual muscle testing of the shoulder shows 5-/5 external rotation and supraspinatus strength, and winging of the right scapula. All other strength tests for the upper extremities are 5/5. Grip strength with a Jamar hand grip dynamometer is 38 kg on the right and 42 on the left. Patient has normal reflexes bilaterally, fully intact light touch sensation in bilateral upper extremities, and negative cervical spine clearing tests.

Active Range of Motion

	Left	Right
Elbow extension	+10	−8
Elbow flexion	145	140
Wrist flexion	80	70
Wrist extension	70	65
Pronation	85	80
Supination	85	85

Assessment of Initial Evaluation

Patient presents with signs and symptoms of lateral humeral epicondylitis with reduced range of motion of the elbow and wrist, and reduced wrist and finger extension strength and a gross reduction of grip strength. The reduction in range of motion of the wrist is consistent with a recent study by Sölveborn and Olerud (1996) of 123 patients with unilateral epicondylitis. Their findings consistently identified reduced wrist flexion and extension active and passive range of motion in the affected extremity.

Initial Treatment and Rehabilitation Goals

The patient's initial treatment consisted of application of electric stimulation to the lateral elbow, gentle passive range of motion and very light stretching particularly of the unaffected muscle tendon units which were measured as inflexible on the initial examination (elbow flexors and forearm pronators). Due to the patient's elbow flexion contracture, a greater emphasis than normal will be placed on flexibility due to the importance of maintaining/achieving full elbow extension to take advantage of the enhanced bony congruity in the fully extended position. Iontophoresis was applied following the treatment directly over the lateral epicondyle. Ice was given to the patient following treatment. She was fit with a counterforce brace to be worn during all tennis activities and during periods of heavy forearm muscle use. She was instructed to modify her teaching activity since completely resting her elbow is not an option due to financial and career obligations. Suggestions to the patient were for use of a ball machine during lessons to rest her elbow and decrease the number of balls that she actually hits, and to limit her tennis playing time as much as possible. She will restring her teaching racquets 2-4 pounds lighter, with respect to string tension, to decrease stress to the forearm and provide greater power with less effort when hitting the ball.

1. Primary initial goal is to decrease lateral elbow pain and encourage healing of the injured tendon by reducing overload stress, modifying activity, and using modalities and anti-inflammatory medication.
2. Following reduction of the initial overload, restoration of complete range of motion and a full return of strength and muscle endurance to the right upper extremity is indicated.

Total Arm Strength Phase

Following four treatments with modalities and light stretching, the patient reports a significant decrease in symptoms, and rates the pain at a 3/10 level with activity and 1/10 at rest. She has not played or competed in tennis and has continued to modify her teaching by using a ball machine. She has demonstrated a tolerance to the initial application of forearm and wrist isotonics with a 2-pound weight, which were initiated on her third treatment as symptoms were decreasing. She also utilizes the upper body ergometer and a complete program of rotator cuff isolation exercises with a 2.5-pound weight. Seated rows, therapeutic ball dribbling, and BOING and *Body Blade* have all been used to encourage a low-resistance, high-repetition resistive exercise approach. Continued use of stretching and joint distraction mobilization has been applied to enhance joint range of motion and muscle tendon unit flexibility. Home program exercise has consisted of the wrist and forearm isotonics, gentle stretching before and after exercise, and generous use of ice. Strict adherence to the suggestions to reduce overload stress to the elbow, including racquet restringing, decreased tennis play, and counterforce brace application have been followed.

Four Weeks Following Initial Treatment

Isokinetic exercise is initiated after four weeks of treatment when the patient can tolerate 5-pound wrist and forearm exercises, and 4-pound rotator cuff exercises prior to the initiation of isokinetic exercise. The pattern of wrist extension/flexion is initially utilized at speeds from 180° to 300° per second. Continued use of the isotonic exercise program as well as the oscillatory and plyometric series of upper extremity exercises attempts to stimulate improved local muscle endurance. Grip strength has improved on the right from 38 on the initial examination to 42 kilograms at this time. Active range of motion of the right elbow is as follows: elbow extension 0°, elbow flexion 0°-140°, wrist flexion 0°-80°, wrist extension 0°-70°, with 85° of pronation and supination of the forearm.

Six Weeks Following Initial Treatment

An isokinetic test is performed which shows wrist flexion, extension, and forearm pronation strength to be 10 percent stronger through the velocity spectrum of 90°, 210°, and 300° per second. Forearm supination strength is equal between extremities. The patient has full elbow extension to 0°, and negative flexion and extension provocation tests bilaterally. The patient is instructed to continue with her exercise program on an alternate day basis and begin the interval tennis program contained on pages 171-172 of this book. Evaluation of the patient's mechanics did identify a backhand technique flaw. The patient was unaware that she had decreased her trunk rotation on her slice backhand, and was using more "arm" to produce force. The patient felt that this may have occurred with teaching as her body fatigued, and carried over into her playing and competitive tennis as well. This is a common fault among players who also teach tennis and feed balls or rally with players for long periods of time. The patient was able to return to competitive tennis without pain, and had a full return of range of motion, muscular strength, and endurance on the right upper extremity kinetic chain from non-operative rehabilitation.

Status Post-Arthroscopic Elbow Debridement

Subjective History

The patient is a 24-year-old left-handed male professional baseball pitcher who is two days status post-arthroscopic debridement and removal of loose bodies, left elbow, April 13, 1994. His initial injury occurred March 16, 1994, during spring training throwing workouts. Patient reports throwing at near-maximal intensities and feeling progressively worsening posterior medial elbow joint pain during the late cocking and acceleration phases of throwing. Symptoms worsened to the point where he was unable to extend his elbow after throwing batting practice. He was sent for orthopedic evaluation and subsequently was found to have osseous irregularities in the posterior medial aspect of his left elbow as well as several loose bodies in the joint. He reports a past history of ulnar collateral ligament sprain that was managed nonoperatively in 1991 during the middle of a season. He was unable to return to 100 percent pitching performance until the beginning of the 1992 season.

Initial Postoperative Findings

The patient has four arthroscopic portal sites that are dry and covered with Steri-Strips. He is fully intact to light touch sensation in dermatomes C5-T1 and has normal vascular filling of the nailbeds of the left hand. Moderate swelling is noted, especially laterally over the radial head, as well as fullness near the olecranon. Palpation of the posterior portal at the triceps tendon reveals a greater amount of scar tissue compared to the other three sites and is slightly more sensitive. There is no significant grinding or crepitus with passive movement, and the patient has a negative radiocapitellar compression test. Ligamentous testing reveals a 1+ valgus stress on the left with a tight endfeel. No medial pain is elicited with this maneuver. The good hands test and Tinel's test are both negative.

Gross Strength Assessment

Jamar handgrip strength is 52 kg on the left and 62 kg on the right, uninjured extremity.

Active Range of Motion

	Left	Right
Elbow extension	-10 °	+2° (hyperextension)
Elbow flexion	130°	140°
Wrist flexion	80°	80°
Wrist extension	65°	75°
Forearm pronation	70°	80°
Forearm supination	70°	90°

Assessment of Initial Evaluation

Mild limitation of elbow extension/flexion range of motion of the left elbow as well as limited wrist extension range of motion. Gross strength (grip) is decreased significantly.

Initial Treatment and Rehabilitation Goals

1. Decrease postoperative pain and swelling using electrical stimulation and ice.
2. Initiate range of motion of the elbow, forearm, and wrist as well as maintain shoulder range of motion. Early use of the upper body ergometer and active-assisted and passive range of motion of the elbow are begun. Accessory mobilization consisting of joint distraction at varying positions of elbow extension/flexion is used.
3. Initiate strengthening of the distal upper extremity. A low-resistance/high-repetition format of strengthening for the elbow extensors and flexors, wrist flexors and extensors, and forearm pronators and supinators is begun using pain-free ranges of motion and no resistance.

4. Recommend home exercise program consisting of continued ice application and use of grip putty, as well as active-assisted range of motion. The patient will be seen three times per week.

Post-Op: One Week

The patient reports minimal pain in the left elbow with ADL activities and continues to deny any neural symptoms. He is pleased with his progression in range of motion and feels that he can extend his elbow further than preoperatively.

Active range of motion, left elbow: +1° of hyperextension to 135° of flexion.

Current treatment protocol: Continued use of modalities to decrease postoperative swelling, with the addition of pulsed ultrasound over the posterior portal due to an increased scar tissue response palpated with examination of the posterior elbow. Soft tissue massage over the portal is also introduced at this time.

Continued range of motion of the shoulder, elbow, forearm, and wrist is carried out, with accessory mobilization via joint distraction being employed.

Additional resistive exercise is begun at this time with isolated rotator cuff work with a 3-pound weight applied proximal to the elbow. Seated rowing and shoulder shrugs are also performed. The patient has progressed to a 3-pound weight with distal isotonic exercises in a pain-free manner. The BOING device for radial/ulnar deviation and pronation/supination movement patterns has been added, along with therapeutic ball dribbling.

Post-Op: Three Weeks

Patient reports no pain with resistive exercise and ADL activity. He feels he is ready to throw and has tried to move his arm through a simulated throwing motion without a ball and has no pain.

Active range of motion, left elbow: +3° of elbow extension to 140° flexion.

Current treatment protocol: Modalities are discontinued in favor of an active warm-up on the upper body ergometer. Range of motion continues for the shoulder, elbow, forearm, and wrist, with discontinuation of accessory mobilization due to the reattainment of active range of motion consistent with the contralateral extremity.

Resistive exercise is progressed, with the patient tolerating a 5-pound weight on distal isotonic exercises. Isokinetic training is introduced using the pattern of wrist flexion/extension at speeds of 180°, 210°, 240°, 270°, and 300° per second. By the end of week 4, the patient is tolerating maximal-level isokinetic wrist extension/flexion and forearm pronation/supination training at fast contractile velocities. Medicine ball plyometrics with

4- and 6-pound balls are initiated at this time. The Plyoback system is used with patterns outlined in this book. Rotator cuff exercises are progressed to 5 pounds, and scapular exercises are continued.

Post-Op: Four Weeks

The patient continues to report no pain with resistive exercises and ADL activities. Clinical examination reveals no areas of palpable tenderness. The triceps arthroscopic portal site is still more prominent than the other three portals but is significantly less prominent than on initial examination. Special tests about the elbow are negative, including the valgus extension overpressure test and the good hands test.

Gross strength: Jamar grip strength is 70 kg on the left, 65 kg on the right.

Isokinetic strength test: Wrist extension/flexion testing shows approximately equal wrist flexion strength bilaterally at speeds of 90°, 210°, and 300° per second for both peak torque and work values. Wrist extension strength is 10 to 15 percent deficient compared to the contralateral extremity. Forearm pronation testing shows 20 to 25 percent greater strength at all three speeds of testing. Forearm supination strength is equal between extremities.

Active range of motion: Elbow extension: +3° of hyperextension, 140° of flexion, 85° of wrist flexion, and 70° of wrist extension, left elbow; 80° of forearm pronation and 90° of forearm supination.

Summary of One-Month Post-Op Evaluation

Complete return of range of motion and improvement of both forearm pronation and wrist extension range of motion. Cybex isokinetic evaluation of wrist strength shows symmetrical strength in wrist flexion, but normative data indicate a normal dominance factor in that muscle group that has resulted in the establishment of a postoperative strength goal of 15 to 20 percent greater strength than on the contralateral extremity. Deficits in wrist extension indicate further need for emphasis in this muscle group. Symmetrical forearm supination strength bilaterally indicates a full return of strength based on normative data for professional baseball pitchers, with greater forearm pronation strength measured on the postoperative extremity at all three testing speeds, again consistent with normative data.

Based on the objective findings in this evaluation, the patient was started at 45 feet on the interval throwing program outlined in this book. He was discharged from formal rehabilitation and placed in direct care of his baseball organization's rehabilitation staff to supervise the progression of the interval throwing program. He continued with twice-weekly visits to physical therapy for isokinetic wrist extension/flexion and forearm pronation/

supination strengthening over the next four weeks. He returned to pitching at the professional level.

Rehabilitation Following Ulnar Nerve Transposition

Subjective History

The patient is an 18-year-old high school baseball pitcher with a one-year history of medial elbow pain. Approximately four months ago, he began having distal paresthesias along the ulnar distribution of the right hand. This pain coincided with the onset of his high school baseball season and continued to worsen during the season, with no improvement in a nonoperative rehabilitation program. Following the season, a four-week rest period also did not diminish the symptoms, which resulted in an ulnar nerve transposition. Postoperatively, the patient reports no neural symptoms in the distal right upper extremity and minimal medial elbow discomfort over the incision. The patient is reporting for his first therapy visit at one week post-op. He is immobilized in a posterior gutter splint, which will be removed during this first therapy visit, and will be fitted with a hinged elbow brace to allow range of motion from -30° to 90°.

Initial Postoperative Findings

Moderate swelling of the medial and posterior aspect of the elbow is noted. The incision is dry and healing well. No ecchymosis is noted. The Tinel's test of the right upper extremity is negative, and there is good distal vascular filling. Further ligamentous and special testing is deferred due to the patient's acute postoperative status.

Active Range of Motion

	Left	Right
Elbow extension	0°	−40°
Elbow flexion	145°	115°
Shoulder flexion	175°	130°
Shoulder abduction	175°	130°
External rotation	90°	45°
Internal rotation	65°	40°

Assessment of Initial Evaluation

Moderate limitation of elbow extension/flexion and shoulder range of motion status post-ulnar nerve transposition.

Initial Rehabilitation Goals and Treatment

Electric stimulation and ice to decrease swelling, gentle range of motion within the range of guidelines (-30° to 100°) using active, passive, and contract-relax PNF stretching techniques. Mobilization and passive stretching to the right shoulder to reduce the capsular pattern of limitation secondary to the period of immobilization of the right upper extremity. Gentle manual resistive exercise for the biceps and triceps in midrange to prevent further disuse atrophy.

Home exercise program: Grip putty for distal strengthening and active-assisted right upper extremity range-of-motion exercise with emphasis on shoulder flexion and abduction.

Post-Op: Three Weeks

Active range of motion of the right elbow is -10° of extension to 140° of flexion. Right shoulder range of motion is 175° of flexion and abduction, with 90° of external rotation and 45° of internal rotation.

Additions to the treatment program have included progression of the patient's extension range of motion during rehabilitation, simultaneously reinforced with advancement of elbow extension range-of-motion stop as per the ulnar nerve protocol and the patient's progress. Upper extremity endurance is addressed by adding the upper body ergometer for 4 to 6 minutes. Initially, a 1-pound weight is used for wrist flexion/extension and pronation/supination resistance. Rotator cuff exercises are initiated, with weight attachment proximal to the elbow. Closed-chain exercises are also added, as well as rhythmic stabilization exercise.

Post-Op: Six Weeks

Active range of motion, right elbow, is -4° of extension to 145° of flexion. Wrist flexion is 80° and bilaterally symmetrical, and wrist extension is 45° (25° less than the contralateral extremity). Grip strength is 35 kg on the left and 29 kg on the right.

Continuation of the patient's range of motion and stretching is followed, with advancement of the distal resistive exercise program to 6 pounds in a controlled manner, with concentric and eccentric muscular emphasis.

Post-Op: Eight Weeks

Active range of motion, right elbow: 0° to 145°.

Isokinetic wrist flexion/extension and forearm pronation/supination isokinetic training are initiated with testing to assess strength. Test results at this time show the right wrist flexors to be 20 to 25 percent stronger at all three test speeds and 10 to 15 percent stronger for wrist extension compared to the left, uninjured extremity. Right forearm pronation strength is 25 to 30 percent greater than the left, and supination strength is equal between extremities.

An interval throwing program was initiated at the 45-foot phase, with continued isokinetic, plyometric, and isotonic training for the entire right upper extremity. The patient continues with rehabilitation, with advancement of the interval throwing program, range-of-motion maintenance, and strength progression.

Post-Op: 12 Weeks

Discharge Evaluation

Range of motion: 0° to 145° of extension/flexion, 0° to 80° of wrist flexion, and 0° to 70° of wrist extension.

Grip strength: 42 kg on the right extremity and 35 kg on the left.

A home exercise program and continued progression of the interval throwing program are given to the patient upon discharge. Throwing off the mound commences upon successful completion of the 150-foot phase of the interval throwing program.

Four-Month Postoperative Follow-Up Evaluation

Range of motion: 0° to 145° of elbow extension/flexion, 0° to 80° of wrist flexion, and 0° to 70° of wrist extension.

Strength: An isokinetic evaluation of the patient at this time shows 30 percent greater wrist flexion strength, 20 percent greater wrist extension strength, 50 to 80 percent greater forearm pronation strength, and 25 percent greater supination strength when compared to the uninjured extremity. The patient has successfully returned to pitching at the competitive level.

Status Post-Ulnar Collateral Ligament Reconstruction Using Autogenous Graft

This case study profiles the progression of an unstable elbow and its ramifications on the surrounding osteochondral structures.

Subjective History

The patient is a 23-year-old right-handed professional baseball pitcher who is status post-ulnar collateral ligament reconstruction using the ipsilateral palmaris longus, with ulnar nerve transposition. The patient is referred for outpatient physical therapy 10 days status postreconstruction. The patient's past musculoskeletal history includes two previous arthroscopic elbow procedures for joint debridement and loose body removal in 1991 and 1994. His most recent arthroscopic surgery (1994) resulted in an initial diminution of posteromedial elbow pain but a return of symptoms upon return to maximal-effort pitching off the mound. Repeated bouts of nonoperative rehabilitation and rest did not allow the patient to continue with maximal-effort performance. Mechanically, the patient reports that he has used an extra "heavy" grip on the ball during the delivery of his curveball, but no other biomechanical changes or modifications are reported relative to his elbow pathology.

Postoperatively, the patient reports minor medial elbow pain and no distal neural symptoms. He has been wearing a posterior splint on the right elbow since surgery.

Initial Postoperative Findings

Minimal swelling is noted in the medial forearm and posterior aspects of the elbow. No ecchymosis is noted, and there is complete closure of the medial elbow incision as well as the small palmar surface forearm incisions used in harvesting the graft. Grip strength is 50 kg on the left extremity and 10 kg on the right. The patient is fully intact to light touch sensation, except for the region immediately surrounding the medial open incision, and the Tinel's test is negative. Shoulder range of motion is limited to 160° of flexion and abduction, but the patient has 90° of external rotation and 35° of internal rotation with 90° of glenohumeral joint abduction.

Active Range of Motion

	Left	Right
Elbow extension	0 °	–65°
Elbow flexion	140°	95°
Wrist flexion	80°	70°
Wrist extension	75°	30°
Forearm pronation	80°	70°
Forearm supination	80°	45°

Assessment of Initial Examination

Good initial range of motion right elbow, with no postoperative neurological compromise in the distal right upper extremity.

Initial Treatment and Rehabilitation Goals

Electric stimulation and ice application to decrease swelling, with early
use of active, passive, and PNF contract-relax stretching for the right elbow, forearm, and wrist. Care is taken not to stretch the wrist flexors and
forearm pronators aggressively due to the recent open medial exposure of
the elbow. Once closure of the medial incision is complete, the patient is
instructed in soft tissue mobilization techniques and gentle cross-friction
massage to mobilize the medial scar. Right shoulder range of motion and
mobilization is used, with care being applied during external rotation
stretching with 90° of abduction due to the stress placed on the medial
elbow in this position. The patient is placed in an elbow immobilizer following treatment, with range-of-motion stops set from -30° to 100° initially.
The patient is given a home exercise program for distal grip strengthening
and active motion within the limits of his elbow brace. The patient is instructed to move the shoulder as much as possible to prevent further disuse and minimize the effects of immobilization.

Post-Op: Two Weeks

With continued range of motion and treatment three times per week, the
patient's range of motion is -20° of elbow extension to 105° of flexion, 90°
of wrist flexion, and 65° of wrist extension. His grip strength has improved
to 22 kg on the right extremity.

Treatment continues on a three-times-per-week basis, with progression
of range of motion per the postoperative protocol and reinforcement of
range-of-motion limitations using the adjustable stops on the brace. Manual

resistance to the elbow, forearm, and wrist is performed, along with light isotonic exercise for wrist extension and forearm supination, and progression into all motions of the forearm and wrist as signs and symptoms allow.

Post-Op: Four Weeks

At one month post-op, the patient has -10° of elbow extension and 120° of flexion. He continues to wear his brace at all times (except during therapy) and has stops set at -10° of extension and 120° of flexion. Light resistance isotonics in all patterns of the distal upper extremity are continued, with ball dribbling, upper body ergometer, and 3-pound isolated rotator cuff exercises with proximal weight attachment.

Post-Op: Eight Weeks

The patient's medial incision is healing well and flattening in appearance, with a gradual reattainment of light touch sensation immediately surrounding the incision. No pain or instability is noted with varus and valgus stress testing of the right elbow when compared bilaterally. Active range of motion is -3° of extension and 135° of flexion, with 90° of wrist flexion and 75° of wrist extension.

Treatment additions during this phase include plyometric upper extremity exercise, 5- to 10-pound distal isotonics, PNF diagonals, and progression of shoulder exercise emphasizing the rotator cuff and scapular musculature. The weight is now placed distal to the elbow at the wrist.

Post-Op: 12 Weeks

Isokinetic wrist extension/flexion exercise is initiated, along with continued distal isotonic and plyometric strengthening. Grip strength is 62 kg on the right extremity and 60 kg on the left. Range of motion of the right elbow continues to be at -3° of extension and 135° flexion.

Post-Op: 16 Weeks

Isokinetic testing of wrist flexion and extension, forearm pronation/supination, and internal/external rotation has been performed. Right wrist flexion strength is approximately equal at 210° and 300° per second between extremities but 10 percent weaker at 90° per second. Wrist extension strength on the right is 15 to 20 percent weaker at 90° and 210° per second but equal at 300° per second. Forearm pronation strength is 10 percent weaker at 90° per second but 15 to 50 percent stronger at the faster testing speeds. An average deficit of 10 percent is found in forearm supination strength.

Consistent strength deficits are identified in the distal muscle groups with slower speeds of testing (90° per second) at this time. Greater muscular tension development may provoke inhibition at this point in the rehabilitation process. Slightly greater overall strength in the pronators, flexors, and extensors is identified at 16 weeks post-op. Testing of the internal and external rotators shows equal external rotation strength bilaterally and 15 to 20 percent greater internal rotation strength on the dominant right upper extremity.

Based on the patient's current range of motion (-3° of extension to 135° of flexion), the lack of pain with resistive testing, and isokinetically documented strength levels, the patient is progressed to an interval throwing program. The initial phase, as outlined in Appendix B, Interval Return Programs: Throwing, begins at 45 feet with a very submaximal intensity. Throwing is initiated on a three-times-per-week basis following a generous warm-up on the upper body ergometer and stretching/mobilization.

Post-Op: Six Months

The patient has progressed through the interval throwing program to the 150-foot level and has started submaximal progression off the mound without pain. He has been throwing off the mound for about three weeks. He presents for a final evaluation of strength and range of motion before reporting for spring training. Isokinetic testing for the shoulder internal and external rotators, wrist flexors and extensors, and forearm pronators and supinators are performed.

Significantly greater external and internal rotation strength is measured at this time on the right shoulder compared to the left at all three testing speeds. Wrist flexion and forearm pronation strength are both significantly stronger on the right arm. Supination strength is approximately equal between extremities, consistent with normative data. Wrist extension strength showed a slight 5 to 10 percent deficit on the right and was a major point of emphasis in the discharge home exercise maintenance program given to the patient during his final visit. Grip strength was measured at 75 kg on the right and 67 kg on the left.

Active range of motion of the right elbow at this time is -2° of elbow extension and 130° of elbow flexion. Wrist flexion is 85° and wrist extension is 55°. Maintenance of forearm and wrist flexibility was emphasized, especially now that greater intensity and frequency of throwing will take place. Valgus stress testing of the right elbow clinically reveals a firm endpoint and less laxity than the contralateral extremity. Light touch sensation and reflexes are normal and bilaterally symmetrical. There is no pain with direct palpation of the medial elbow. The patient was formally discharged from physical therapy and is under the direct supervision of the training staff of his baseball team.

Status Post-Open Reduction Internal Fixation Medial Epicondylar Growth Plate

Subjective History

The patient is a right-handed 16-year-old male high school baseball pitcher who is status post-open reduction internal fixation of a medial epicondylar growth plate fracture, March 31, 1994. This patient initially injured his elbow March 24, 1994, pitching in a high school baseball game. He reports feeling a popping sensation in the medial aspect of his right elbow during the acceleration phase. He was unable to continue throwing and had pain with activities that extended his elbow as well as those that produced a valgus stress about the elbow.

He reports to the clinic in an elbow immobilizer locked in 90° of elbow flexion, which he has worn continuously for three weeks since the surgery. He reports minimal pain at the present time and denies any distal paresthesias. He is not taking any medications and reports no previous injury to the right elbow but has a history of right shoulder tendinitis in the fall of 1993.

Initial Postoperative Findings

A well-healed medial incision of approximately 3.5 to 4 inches is noted. There is a slight decrease in light touch sensation in the immediate medial and lateral margins of the operative incision. The Tinel's test is negative, and no thickening is noted with palpation of the ulnar nerve. There is normal vascular filling of the fingertips and symmetrical light touch sensation of the entire upper extremity, except for the region noted above. No tenderness is elicited with palpation over the bony and soft tissue landmarks about the elbow. Valgus stress testing of the elbow is not performed at this time due to the patient's acute postoperative nature. No significant grinding is noted with passive motion of the elbow and radioulnar joints, and a radiocapitellar compression test is negative.

Gross Strength Assessment

Jamar hand grip strength shows 42 kg on the uninjured left extremity and 40 kg on the right, dominant extremity. Manual muscle testing of the elbow extensors and flexors is 5-/5, forearm supination and wrist extension is 5/5, and wrist flexion and forearm pronation is 4/5. All measures on the left, uninjured extremity are 5/5.

Active Range of Motion

	Left	Right
Elbow extension	0 °	–55°
Elbow flexion	145°	120°
Wrist flexion	60°	55°
Wrist extension	55°	55°
Forearm pronation	90°	80°
Forearm supination	90°	70°
Radial deviation	30°	30°
Ulnar deviation	20°	20°
Shoulder flexion	170°	150°
Shoulder abduction	170°	145°
Shoulder external rotation	90°	70°
Shoulder internal rotation	70°	35°

Assessment of Initial Evaluation

Moderate limitation of elbow extension range of motion with shoulder motion loss secondary to immobilization of the right upper extremity post-op. Decrease in distal grip strength and specific loss of manually assessed forearm pronation and wrist flexion strength.

Initial Treatment and Rehabilitation Goals

Electrical stimulation to the right elbow, with active-assisted and PNF contract-relax range-of-motion techniques for the right elbow to improve elbow extension range of motion. General elbow joint mobilization using joint distraction in varying positions of elbow extension/flexion. Shoulder mobilization and passive stretching to reduce the capsular pattern of range-of-motion limitation secondary to immobilization. Submaximal manual resistance to the distal upper extremity to begin contracting the musculature surrounding the elbow.

Initial home exercise program: Shoulder and elbow active-assisted range of motion; therapy putty for distal grip strengthening.

Initial rehab frequency: Three times per week with twice-daily home exercise execution.

Post-Op: Four Weeks

After one month post-op, the patient has now received three sessions of physical therapy. Since the first three weeks post-op, the patient has been immobilized in 90° of elbow flexion without physical therapy.

Active range of motion: -15° of elbow extension to 140° of elbow flexion. Shoulder active range of motion is bilaterally symmetrical at 170° of flexion and abduction and 90° of external rotation with 90° abduction. Internal rotation of the dominant right shoulder is 55°.

Current treatment protocol: Continued use of modalities prior to mobilization and stretching of the elbow, forearm, and wrist. Use of the upper body ergometer has been initiated, as well as 1.5-pound distal isotonics exercise using the patterns of elbow extension/flexion, wrist extension/flexion, radial/ulnar deviation, and forearm pronation/supination. Manual resistance of elbow extension/flexion is used via a pain-free range of motion. Ball dribbling has been added using therapeutic balls and shoulder scaption and prone extension/horizontal abduction with proximal weight attachment of 3 pounds. Proprioceptive training without visual assistance using joint angular replication is used due to the medial incision and possible afferent neural feedback damage. Several angles within the patient's comfortable range of motion are used.

Home exercise additions include wrist extension/flexion and forearm pronation/supination with surgical tubing (red Thera-Band level); radial/ulnar deviation with a counterbalanced weight such as a hammer or tennis racquet.

Post-Op: Eight Weeks

Active range of motion, right elbow: -5° of extension to 140° of flexion.

Current treatment protocol: Discontinuation of modalities, with continued use of elbow joint mobilization to promote elbow extension, such as joint distraction toward end ranges of elbow extension to stress the anterior capsule, passive and active-assisted stretching of the elbow forearm and wrist, and progression of the isotonic distal strengthening program to 5 pounds. Additional exercises at this time are introduction of the patient to isokinetic wrist extension/flexion at speeds of 180° to 300° per second and plyometric medicine ball tosses using a 6-pound ball. Resistive internal and external rotation to the shoulder as well as serratus and rowing exercise to address the scapular stabilizers have been used over the past two weeks.

Post-Op: 12 Weeks

Active range of motion, right arm: -2° of elbow extension and 145° of elbow flexion, 79° of wrist flexion and 55° of wrist extension, 30° of radial deviation, and 20° of ulnar deviation.

Grip strength: 50 kg on the right extremity, 45 kg on the left.

Isokinetic strength testing: The patient underwent an isokinetic strength test for wrist extension/flexion, forearm pronation/supination, and elbow extension/flexion. Results of the testing show symmetrical strength in wrist extension and forearm supination, as well as in elbow extension/flexion. Ten to 15 percent deficits are still present in the forearm pronators and wrist flexors of the dominant right extremity when compared bilaterally.

Discharge Plan

The patient was reinstructed in the distal isotonic exercises with progression to 10 pounds, with a high-repetition goal being planned. Rubber tubing was prescribed for wrist flexion/extension and shoulder internal/external rotation at more advanced levels of resistance. The interval throwing program is to be initiated starting at 45 feet, with the recommendation that the patient remain at this level for two weeks due to the presence of wrist flexor and forearm pronator weakness that was documented objectively with isokinetic testing. Progression of the interval program is to be followed until the patient can throw 120 feet in a pain-free manner repetitively. At that point, the patient has been instructed to return to throwing off the mound at 50 percent effort. The patient was given a flexibility program for the upper extremity with particular emphasis on continued improvement of elbow extension range of motion. Shoulder internal rotation stretches were also given due to the limitation of that range, even with mobilization and stretching performed in therapy.

Postoperative Protocols

Tennis Elbow

Days 1-7

a. Expect a good bit of soreness.

b. Keep elbow immobilized the majority of time.

c. Sleep if possible on back with arm on pillow on stomach.

d. Be sure to keep full shoulder motion and move shoulder fully several times each day.

e. Days 1-3, the elbow should stay bandaged and in the immobilizer at all times.

f. Starting about day 2: move fingers and wrist for 2 minutes, 3-5X/day.

g. You may shower on the third day after surgery: remove bandages, gently work the elbow in the shower. After showering, gently air or blow-dry the wound then cleanse gently with alcohol and cover the wound with bandaids.

h. Days 3-6, wear the immobilizer at all times except for shower and gently limbering the elbow.

i. Ice several times a day for 20-30 minutes at a time.

j. Medications: Use pain or anti-inflammatory medications as prescribed by your doctor. If you are taking no anti-inflammatory medicine you may take aspirin or Tylenol. **Do not take aspirin and anti-inflammatory medicine simultaneously.**

Expect significant deep elbow pain through the next weeks. This reflects the work done and the healing process!!!

Recheck With Your Doctor If

• The wound looks "angry"—excessive swelling, dramatically increased pain which progressively worsens

• Increased fever

Days 7-17

    a. Limber your elbow with bending and straightening motions. Start in warm shower.

    b. By day 17 about 80% of elbow motion return is average.

    c. Work on wrist, fingers, forearm pronation and supination (active motion).

    d. Use arm for light activities.

    e. Use immobilizer occasionally for protection only. Leave immobilizer off the majority of the time.

Days 17-21

    a. Use counterforce brace with light tension when exercising.

    b. Begin squeezing a Nerf ball.

    c. Actively bend and straighten elbow through fullest possible range.

    d. Do tennis elbow exercises as prescribed by your therapist or doctor without any weight. Start with 5 repetitions, work up to 15 repetitions of each.

Three Weeks

    a. Begin full tennis elbow exercise program including light weights—use counterforce brace with comfortable tension.

    b. Increase use of arm over 3-6 week period for normal activities.

    c. Relief of pre-surgery pain is usually noted in the 3-6 week period. Maintain as high a level of aerobic activity as you did preoperatively (e.g., jogging, etc.). If you note increased pain you may have overstressed the arm:

        • Use ice as needed for 20 minutes on, 20 minutes off to relieve pain

        • Decrease your activity level.

On average your arm will return to normal in _____ months. However, there may be occasions over the next year where you experience discomfort. Use ice, aspirin, Tylenol or Advil at these times. Contact your doctor if major pain lasts more than 3 days.

Data from Robert P. Nirschl, MD, Virginia Sports Medicine Institute, Arlington, VA.

Elbow Arthroscopy and Removal of Loose Bodies

Post-Op Days 1 & 2
  a. Removal of bulky post-op dressing and replacement with Ace wrap
  b. Electric stimulation and ice to decrease pain/inflammation
  c. Initiation of range-of-motion exercise for the glenohumeral joint, elbow, forearm, and wrist
  d. Initiation of sub-maximal strengthening exercises including:
    1. putty
    2. isometric elbow and wrist flexion/extension
    3. isometric forearm pronation/supination

Post-Op Days 2-7
  a. Range of motion and joint mobilization to terminal ranges for the elbow, forearm, and wrist. (Avoid over-aggressive elbow extension passive range of motion.)
  b. Begin progressive resistance exercise program with 0 to 1 pound weight and three sets of 15 repetitions
    1. wrist flexion curls
    2. wrist extension curls
    3. radial deviation
    4. ulnar deviation
    5. forearm pronation
    6. forearm supination
  c. Upper body ergometer

Post-Op Days 7-3 Weeks
  a. Continue progressive resistance exercise program adding:
    1. elbow extension
    2. elbow flexion
    3. isolated rotator cuff program (Jobe exercises)
    4. seated row
    5. manual and isotonic scapular program
    6. closed chain upper extremity program

Post-Op 4-6 Weeks
  a. Isokinetic exercise introduction using wrist flexion/extension and forearm pronation/supination movement patterns
  b. Upper extremity plyometrics with medicine balls
  c. Isokinetic test to formally assess distal strength
  d. Interval Sport Return Program

1. Criteria for advancement:
   a. full, pain-free range of motion
   b. (85-100) percent return of muscle strength
   c. no provocation of pain on clinical exam
   e. Upper extremity strength and flexibility maintenance program

Ulnar Nerve Transposition

General Guidelines

- Physician rechecks at 1, 2, 6, and 12 weeks post-op.
- Do not exercise through specific joint pain.

Post-Op Week 1

a. Patient immobilized in posterior splint/brace, in 90° of elbow flexion.

b. Modalities as indicated to decrease swelling, pain, and inflammation.

c. AROM and PROM -30° extension to 100° of flexion postoperative elbow.

d. ROM into wrist flexion and forearm pronation with guarded ROM for wrist extension and forearm supination to protect flexor/pronator origin postoperatively.

e. Ball/putty squeezes for grip strengthening.

f. Isometric elbow extension/flexion, wrist extension/flexion, and radial/ulnar deviation.

Post-Op Week 2

a. Patient immobilized in brace, with limitations to last 15° of elbow extension.

b. AROM and PROM continue, using a range of -15° of elbow extension to 120° of elbow flexion.

c. Strengthening continues, using isometric and light isotonic exercises for elbow extension/flexion, wrist flexion/extension, forearm pronation/supination, and wrist radial/ulnar deviation in a pain-free ROM. Emphasis on low resistance, with 3 sets of 15 reps each pattern.

d. Upper body ergometer as tolerated.

Post-Op Week 3

a. ROM progressed to terminal ranges as tolerated, with respect to elbow extension/flexion.

b. Strengthening continues with isotonic exercise.

Post-Op Week 4

a. Scapular and shoulder strenthening exercises are commenced with point of resistance application being proximal to the elbow, to minimize stress across the elbow joint.

Post-Op Week 8
 a. Initiation of isokinetic wrist flexion/extension and forearm prona-
   tion/supination submaximal exercise as tolerated.
  • Criterion for progression of isokinetic exercise:
   – Full ROM of the wrist and forearm.
   – Tolerance of isotonic strengthening procedures.

Post-Op Week 10-12
 a. Isokinetic evaluation to formally assess wrist flexion/extension and
   forearm pronation/supination strength.
 b. Physician evaluation to assess progression to functional return in
   interval sport programs.

Ulnar Collateral Ligament Reconstruction Using Autogenous Graft (Seto et al. 1991)

Time Period (postoperation)	Exercise Program
0 to 1/2 mo.	Elbow immobilized. Gripping exercises.
1/2 to 1 mo.	Splint removed. PROM and active-assisted elbow ROM. Active shoulder ROM exercises (if necessary).
1 to 1 1/2 mos.	Active elbow and shoulder ROM exercises. Strengthening exercises: wrist flexion and extension, forearm pronation and supination.
1 1/2 to 3 mos.	Continue shoulder and elbow ROM exercises. Continue wrist and forearm strengthening exercises. Add elbow strengthening exercises. May add resistive radial and ulnar deviation.
3 to 5 mos.	Avoid valgus stress to elbow and ballistic movement in terminal elbow ranges. May begin shoulder strengthening exercises with light resistance, with emphasis on rotator cuff muscles. Start total body conditioning exercises. May begin easy tossing at 30 feet, progressing to 50 feet, no wind-up, 2-3 times/week, 10-15 min/session.
5 to 5 1/2 mos.	Continue upper extremity strengthening exercises. Continue easy tossing, 50-60 feet, no wind-up, 2-3 times/week, 10-15 min/session.
5 1/2 to 6 mos.	Add shoulder internal rotation exercise in sidelying position. Continue strengthening exercises and total body conditioning program. Lob ball on alternate days, no more than 30 feet, 10-15 min/session.
6 to 6 1/2 mos.	Lob with easy wind-up, 40-50 feet, 15-20 min/session, 2-3 times/week.
6 1/2 to 7 mos.	Lob with occasional straight throw at 1/2 speed, 60 feet, 20-25 min/session, 2-3 times/week.

(continued)

(continued)

Time Period (postoperation)	Exercise Program
7 to 7 1/2 mos.	Increase throwing distance to 100 feet at 1/2 speed, 20-25 min/session, 2-3 times/week
7 1/2 to 8 mos.	Long easy throws from 150 feet with ball back to home plate on 5-6 bounces, 20-25 min/session. Begin 12-Day Throwing Cycle: Throw 2 days/rest one day, repeat 4 times.
8 to 8 1/2 mos.	**Outfielders:** Increase throwing distance to 200-250 feet, with ball reaching home plate on numerous bounces, 20-25 min/session, 12-Day Throwing Cycle. **Pitchers and infielders:** In and Out Drill: Begin throwing at 3/4 speed, gradually increasing the throwing distance until 150 feet. Gradually decrease throwing distance until reaching normal throwing position distance. Perform this drill 30-35 minutes on the 12-Day Throwing Cycle.
8 1/2 to 9 mos.	**Outfielders:** Increase throwing distance to 300-350 feet, with ball reaching home plate on 1-2 bounces at 3/4 speed-full speed, 30-35 min/session, 12-Day Throwing Cycle. **Pitchers and infielders:** In and Out Drill: Gradually reduce time throwing "in and out" and increase throwing time from normal playing position, 3/4 speed-full speed, 30-35 min/session, 12-Day Throwing Cycle.
9 to 9 1/2 mos.	**Outfielders and infielders:** Short, crisp throws from 100-150 feet, 3/4-full speed, 30 minutes, 12-Day Throwing Cycle. **Pitchers:** Throw batting practice at 3/4-full speed, 30 minutes, 12-Day Throwing Cycle.
9 1/2 to 10 1/2 mos.	**All players:** Return to throwing from normal playing position, 3/4-full speed with emphasis on technique and accuracy, 25-30 min/session, 12-Day Throwing Cycle.
10 1/2 to 11 mos.	**All players:** Continue throwing from normal playing position, 7/8-full speed, gradually increase throwing time.
11 to 12 mos.	**All players:** Simulate game day situation. **Pitchers:** Warm up with appropriate number of pitches and throw for an average number of innings, taking the usual rest breaks between innings. Repeat this simulation 2-4 times with a 3-4 day rest period in between.

Chronic Ulnar Collateral Ligament Reconstruction Using Autogenous Graft (Wilk et al. 1995)

Phase I: Immediate postoperative phase (0-3 weeks)
Goals:
- Protect healing tissue
- Decrease pain/inflammation
- Retard muscular atrophy
a. Postoperative week 1
- Posterior splint at 90° elbow flexion
- Wrist AROM ext/flexion
- Elbow compression dressing (2-3 days)
- Exercises: gripping exercises, wrist range of motion (ROM), shoulder isometrics (except shoulder ER), biceps isometrics
- Cryotherapy
b. Postoperative week 2
- Application of functional brace 30-100°
- Initiate wrist isometrics
- Initiate elbow flex/ext isometrics
- Continue all exercises listed above
c. Postoperative week 3
- Advance brace 15-110°, gradually increase ROM; 5° extension/10° flexion per week

Phase II: Intermediate phase (weeks 4-8)
Goals:
- Gradual increase in ROM
- Promote healing of repaired tissue
- Regain and improve muscular strength
a. Week 4
- Functional brace set (10-120°)
- Begin light resistance exercises for arm (1 lb): wrist curls, extensions, pronation/supination, elbow ext/flexion
- Progress shoulder program, emphasize rotator cuff strengthening (avoid ER until 6th week)
b. Week 6
- Functional brace set (0-130°); active range of motion (AROM) 0-145° (without brace)
- Progress elbow strengthening exercises
- Initiate shoulder external rotation strengthening
- Progress shoulder program

Phase III: Advanced strengthening phase (weeks 9-13)
Goals:
- Increase strength, power, endurance
- Maintain full elbow ROM
- Gradually initiate sporting activities

a. Week 9
- Initiate eccentric elbow flexion/extension
- Continue isotonic program; forearm and wrist
- Continue shoulder program—Throwers Ten Program
- Manual resistance diagonal patterns
- Initiate plyometric exercise program

b. Week 11
- Continue all exercises listed above
- May begin light sport activities (i.e., golf, swimming)

Phase IV: Return to activity phase (weeks 14-26)
Goals:
- Continue to increase strength, power, and endurance of upper extremity musculature
- Gradual return to sport activities

a. Week 14
- Initiate interval throwing program (phase I)
- Continue strengthening program
- Emphasis on elbow and wrist strengthening and flexibility exercises

b. Week 22-26
- Return to competitive throwing

Interval Return Programs

Tennis

Begin at stage indicated by your therapist or doctor.

Do not progress or continue program if joint pain is present.

Always stretch your shoulder, elbow, and wrist before and after the interval program.

Ice after completion of the program.

Do not use a backboard for the interval program, because it leads to exaggerated muscle work, without rest between strokes.

It is highly recommended that your strokes be evaluated by a USPTA certified teaching professional.

Play on alternate days, giving your body a recovery day between sessions.

Preliminary Stage: Foam ball impact, beginning with ball feeds from the net from partner. 20-25 forehands and backhands only.

Perform each stage _____ times before progressing to the next stage. Do not progress to the next phase if pain or excessive fatigue was present during your last outing.

Stage 1: a. Have a partner feed 20 forehand groundstrokes from the net (feeds should be looping and waist high).

b. Have a partner feed 20 backhand groundstrokes from the net, as in 1a above.

c. Rest 5 minutes.

d. Repeat 20 forehands and backhands from ball feeds.

Stage 2: a. Begin as in Stage 1 above, with partner feeding 20 forehands and backhands from the net.

b. Rally with a partner from the baseline, hitting controlled groundstrokes, mixing both forehands and backhands for 50-60 repetitions.

c. Rest 5 minutes.

d. Repeat 2b above.

Stage 3: a. Rally groundstrokes from the baseline for 15 minutes.

b. Rest 5 minutes.

c. Hit 10 forehand and backhand volleys, emphasizing a contact point in front of your body.

d. Rally 15 minutes from the baseline.

e. Hit 10 forehand and backhand volleys.

_____**Pre-Serve Interval** (perform prior to Stage 4)

a. After stretching with racquet in hand, perform serving motion 10-15 times, without a ball.

b. Using a foam ball, hit 10-15 serves without concern for performance result (only form of racquet arm and contact point).

Stage 4: a. Hit 20 minutes of groundstrokes, mixing in volleys using a 70% groundstroke/30% volley format.

b. Hit 10 serves.

c. Rest 5 minutes.

d. Hit 10-15 more serves.

e. Finish with 5-10 minutes of groundstrokes.

Stage 5: a. Repeat stages 4a and 4b listed above, increasing the number of serves to 20-25 instead of 10-15.

b. Before resting, have a partner feed easy short lobs to attempt a controlled overhead smash. Repeat overhead 5-10 repetitions.

c. Finish as in Stage 4 above, with 5-10 minutes of groundstrokes.

Stage 6: Prior to attempting match play, complete steps 1-5 without pain or excess fatigue in the upper extremity. Do not progress from stage to stage if pain develops.

Throwing for Baseball Players

General Guidelines

The Interval Throwing Program (ITP) is designed to gradually return motion, strength, and confidence in the throwing arm after injury or surgery by slowly progressing through graduated throwing distances.

• **Weight Training.** The athlete should supplement the ITP with a high-repetition, low-weight exercise program. Strengthening should address a good balance between anterior and posterior musculature so that the shoulder will not be predisposed to injury. Special emphasis must be given to posterior rotator cuff musculature for any strengthening program.

• **Individual Variability.** The ITP is designed so that each level is achieved without pain or complication before the next level is started. This sets up a progression that a goal is achieved prior to advancement instead of advancing to a specific time frame. Because of this design, the ITP may be used for different levels of skills and abilities from those in high school to professional levels.

• **Warm-up.** Jogging increases blood flow to the muscles and joints thus increasing their flexibility and decreasing the chance of reinjury. Since the amount of warm-up will vary from person to person, the athlete should jog until developing a light sweat, then progress to the stretching phase.

• **Stretching.** Since throwing involves all muscles in the body; all muscle groups should be stretched prior to throwing. This should be done in a systematic fashion beginning with the legs and including the trunk, back, neck, and arms.

• **Throwing Mechanics.** A critical aspect of the ITP is maintenance of proper throwing mechanics through the advancement.

• **Summary.** In using the Interval Throwing Program (ITP) in conjunction with a structured rehabilitation program, the athlete should be able to return to full competition status, minimizing any chance of reinjury. The program and its progression should be modified to meet the specific needs of each individual athlete. A comprehensive program consisting of a maintenance strength and flexibility program, appropriate warm-up and cool-down procedures, proper pitching mechanics, and progressive throwing and batting will assist the baseball player in returning safely to competition.

Phase I: Initial Throwing

45' Phase
Step 1: a. Warm-up throwing
       b. 45' (25 throws)
       c. Rest 15 minutes
       d. Warm-up throwing
       e. 45' (25 throws)
Step 2: a. Warm-up throwing
       b. 45' (25 throws)
       c. Rest 10 minutes
       d. Warm-up throwing
       e. 45' (25 throws)
       f. Rest 10 minutes
       g. Warm-up throwing
       h. 45' (25 throws)

60' Phase
Step 3: a. Warm-up throwing
       b. 60' (25 throws)
       c. Rest 15 minutes
       d. Warm-up throwing
       e. 60' (25 throws)
Step 4: a. Warm-up throwing
       b. 60' (25 throws)
       c. Rest 10 minutes
       d. Warm-up throwing
       e. 60' (25 throws)
       f. Rest 10 minutes
       g. Warm-up throwing
       h. 60' (25 throws)

90' Phase
Step 5: a. Warm-up throwing
       b. 90' (25 throws)
       c. Rest 15 minutes
       d. Warm-up throwing
       e. 90' (25 throws)
Step 6: a. Warm-up throwing
       b. 90' (25 throws)
       c. Rest 10 minutes
       d. Warm-up throwing
       e. 90' (25 throws)
       f. Rest 10 minutes
       g. Warm-up throwing
       h. 90' (25 throws)

120' Phase
Step 7: a. Warm-up throwing
       b. 120' (25 throws)
       c. Rest 15 minutes
       d. Warm-up throwing
       e. 120' (25 throws)
Step 8: a. Warm-up throwing
       b. 120' (25 throws)
       c. Rest 10 minutes
       d. Warm-up throwing
       e. 120' (25 throws)
       f. Rest 10 minutes
       g. Warm-up throwing
       h. 120' (25 throws)

150' Phase
Step 9: a. Warm-up throwing
       b. 150' (25 throws)
       c. Rest 15 minutes
       d. Warm-up throwing
       e. 150' (25 throws)
Step 10: a. Warm-up throwing
       b. 150' (25 throws)
       c. Rest 10 minutes
       d. Warm-up throwing
       e. 150' (25 throws)
       f. Rest 10 minutes
       g. Warm-up throwing
       h. 150' (25 throws)

180' Phase
Step 11: a. Warm-up throwing
       b. 180' (25 throws)
       c. Rest 15 minutes
       d. Warm-up throwing
       e. 180' (25 throws)
Step 12: a. Warm-up throwing
       b. 180' (25 throws)
       c. Rest 10 minutes
       d. Warm-up throwing
       e. 180' (25 throws)
       f. Rest 10 minutes

g. Warm-up throwing
h. 180' (25 throws)

Step 13: a. Warm-up throwing
b. 180' (25 throws)
c. Rest 10 minutes
d. Warm-up throwing
e. 180' (25 throws)

f. Rest 10 minutes
g. Warm-up throwing
h. 180' (50 throws)

Step 14: Begin throwing off the mound or return to respective position.

Phase II: Starting Off the Mound

Stage One: Fastball Only

Step 1: Interval throwing
15 Throws off mound 50%

Step 2: Interval throwing
30 Throws off mound 50%

Step 3: Interval throwing
45 Throws off mound 50%

Step 4: Interval throwing
60 Throws off mound 50%

Step 5: Interval throwing
30 Throws off mound 75%

Step 6: 30 Throws off mound 75%
45 Throws off mound 50%

Step 7: 45 Throws off mound 75%
15 Throws off mound 50%

Step 8: 60 Throws off mound 75%

Stage Two: Fastball Only

Step 9: 45 Throws off mound 75%
15 Throws in batting practice

Step 10: 45 Throws off mound 75%
30 Throws in batting practice

Step 11: 45 Throws off mound 75%
45 Throws in batting practice

Stage Three

Step 12: 30 Throws off mound 75% warm-up
15 Throws off mound 50% breaking balls
45-60 Throws in batting practice (fastball only)

Step 13: 30 Throws off mound 75%
30 Breaking balls 75%
30 Throws in batting practice

Step 14: 30 Throws off mound 75%
60-90 Throws in batting practice 25% breaking balls

Step 15: Simulated game:
Progressing by 15 throws per work-out

Little Leaguer Interval Throwing Program

The little leaguer interval throwing program parallels the interval throwing program in returning the little leaguer to a graduated progression of throwing distances. Warm-up and stretching should be performed prior to throwing.

30' Phase

Step 1: a. Warm-up throwing
        b. 30' (25 throws)
        c. Rest 15 minutes
        d. Warm-up throwing
        e. 30' (25 throws)

Step 2: a. Warm-up throwing
        b. 30' (25 throws)
        c. Rest 10 minutes
        d. Warm-up throwing
        e. 30' (25 throws)
        f. Rest 10 minutes
        g. Warm-up throwing
        h. 30' (25 throws)

45' Phase

Step 3: a. Warm-up throwing
        b. 45' (25 throws)
        c. Rest 15 minutes
        d. Warm-up throwing
        e. 45' (25 throws)

Step 4: a. Warm-up throwing
        b. 45' (25 throws)
        c. Rest 10 minutes
        d. Warm-up throwing
        e. 45' (25 throws)
        f. Rest 10 minutes
        g. Warm-up throwing
        h. 45' (25 throws)

60' Phase

Step 5: a. Warm-up throwing
        b. 60' (25 throws)
        c. Rest 15 minutes
        d. Warm-up throwing
        e. 60' (25 throws)

Step 6: a. Warm-up throwing
        b. 60' (25 throws)
        c. Rest 10 minutes
        d. Warm-up throwing
        e. 60' (25 throws)
        f. Rest 10 minutes
        g. Warm-up throwing
        h. 60' (25 throws)

90' Phase

Step 7: a. Warm-up throwing
        b. 90' (25 throws)
        c. Rest 15 minutes
        d. Warm-up throwing
        e. 90' (25 throws)

Step 8: a. Warm-up throwing
        b. 90' (25 throws)
        c. Rest 10 minutes
        d. Warm-up throwing
        e. 90' (25 throws)
        f. Rest 10 minutes
        g. Warm-up throwing
        h. 90' (25 throws)

Data from Wilk, K.E. & Andrews, J.R., American Sports Medicine Institute, Birmingham, AL.

Golf

General Guidelines

- Perform flexibility exercises before hitting, and use ice after play.
- Chips should be performed with a pitching wedge.
- Short irons are W, 9, 8; medium irons, 7, 6, 5; long irons, 4, 3, 2; woods, 3, 5.
- Drives should be performed with a driver.

Week	Day of Week		
	Monday	**Wednesday**	**Friday**
1	10 putts	15 putts	20 putts
	10 chips	15 chips	20 chips
	5-min rest	5-min rest	5-min rest
	15 chips	25 chips	20 putts
			20 chips
			5-min rest
			10 chips
			10 short irons
2	20 chips	20 chips	15 short irons
	10 short irons	15 short irons	10 medium irons
	5-min rest	10-min rest	10-min rest
	10 short irons	15 short irons	20 short irons
		15 chips putting	15 chips
3	15 short irons	15 short irons	15 short irons
	15 medium irons	10 medium irons	10 medium irons
	10-min rest	10 long irons	10 long irons
	5 long irons	10-min rest	10-min rest
	15 short irons	10 short irons	10 short irons
	15 medium irons	10 medium irons	10 medium irons
	10-min rest	5 long irons	10 long irons
	20 chips	5 wood	10 wood
4	15 short irons	9 holes	9 holes
	10 medium irons		
	10 long irons		
	10 drives		
	15-min rest		
	Repeat		
5	9 holes	9 holes	18 holes

Adapted from Wilk et al. 1995.

100-Point Classification System for Clinical Outcomes

Categories	Definition	Point Values
Pain	None	45
	Mild	30
	Moderate	15
	Severe	0
Motion	Arc > 100 degrees	20
	Arc > 50-100 degrees	15
	Arc < 50 degrees	5
Stability	Stable	10
	Moderate Instability	5
	Gross Instability	0
Function	Combing hair	5
(25 points total)	Eating	5
	Washing	5
	Putting on shirt	5
	Putting on shoes	5

Clinical outcome: Excellent > 90, Good 75-89, Fair 60-74, Poor < 60

Data from Morrey 1993.

Credits

Figure 2.1 Reprinted, by permission, from W.B. Leadbetter, J.B. Buckwalter, and S.L. Gordon (Eds.), 1990, *Sports-induced inflammation: Clinical and basic science concepts* (Park Ridge, IL: American Academy of Orthopaedic Surgeons), 2.

Figure 2.2 Reprinted, by permission, from W.B. Leadbetter, 1992, "Cell matrix response in tendon injury," *Clinics in Sports Medicine* 11(3): 537.

Figure 2.4 Adapted, by permission, from P.A. Indelicato et al., 1979, "Correctable elbow lesions in professional baseball players," *American Journal of Sports Medicine* 7(1): 72-75.

Figure 3.1 Photo courtesy of Austin & Associates, Fallston, MD.

Figure 6.14 and 6.15 Adapted from B.F. Morrey, 1994, The elbow. In *Master techniques in orthopedic surgery series*, edited by R.C. Thompson (New York: Raven Press).

Figure 6.16, 6.17, 6.18, and 6.20 and Table 6.1 Reprinted, by permission, from J.R. Andrews and S.R. Soffer, 1994, *Elbow arthroscopy* (St. Louis: Mosby-Year Book, Inc.).

Figure 6.19 Reprinted, by permission, from J.C. Esch and C.L. Baker, 1993, *Arthroscopic surgery: The shoulder and the elbow* (Philadelphia: J.B. Lippincott).

Figure 6.23 Adapted, by permission, from Jobe and Elattrache, 1993, Diagnosis and treatment of ulnar collateral ligament injuries in athletes. In *The elbow and its disorders*, edited by B.F. Morrey (Philadelphia: W.B. Saunders), 570.

Photo on page 110 courtesy of Joint Solutions, Tustin, CA.

Photo on page 111 courtesy of Prince and Ektelon Sports Group.

Interval Golf Program (Appendix B, page 177) Adapted, with permission, from K.E. Wilk, F.M. Azar, and J.R. Andrews, 1995, "Conservative and operative rehabilitation of the elbow in sports," *Sports Medicine and Arthroscopy Review* 3(3): 253.

References

Adams, J.E. (1968). Bone injuries in very young athletes. *Clinical Ortho-paedics, 58*, 129.

Adelsberg, S. (1986). An EMG analysis of selected muscles with rackets of increasing grip size. *American Journal of Sports Medicine, 14*, 139-142..

Albright, J.A., Jokl, P., Shaw, R., & Albright, J.P. (1978). Clinical study of baseball pitchers: Correlation of injury to the throwing arm with method of delivery. *American Journal of Sports Medicine, 6*, 15-21.

An, K.N., Hui, F.C., Morrey, B.F., Linscheid, R.L., & Chao, E.Y. (1981). Muscles across the elbow joint: A biomechanical analysis. *Journal of Biomechanics, 14*, 659-669.

An, K.N., & Morrey, B.F. (1993). Biomechanics of the elbow. In B.F. Morrey, *The elbow and its disorders* (2nd ed.) (pp. 53-72). Philadelphia: W.B. Saunders.

Anderson, M.A., & Rutt, R.A. (1992). The effects of counterforce bracing on wrist and forearm muscle function. *Journal of Orthopaedic and Sports Physical Therapy, 15*(2), 87-91.

Andrews, J.R. (1985). Bony injuries about the elbow in the throwing athlete. In Instructional Course Lectures, *Injuries of the upper extremity in the competitive athlete, 34*, 323-331. Rosemont, IL: American Academy of Orthopaedic Surgeons.

Andrews, J.R., & Craven, W.M. (1991). Lesions of the posterior compartment of the elbow. *Clinics in Sports Medicine, 10*, 637-652.

Andrews, J.R., & Frank, W. (1985). Valgus extension overload in the pitching elbow. In J.R. Andrews, B. Zarins, & W.B. Carson (Eds.), *Injuries to the throwing arm* (pp. 250-257). Philadelphia: W.B. Saunders.

Andrews, J.R., & McKenzie, P.J. (1991). Arthroscopic surgical treatment of elbow pathology. In J.B. McGinty (Ed.), *Operative arthroscopy* (p. 595). New York: Raven.

Andrews, J.R., & Soffer, S.R. (1994). *Elbow arthroscopy*. St. Louis: Mosby Year Book Inc.

Andrews, J.R., St. Pierre, R.K., & Carson, W.G. (1986). Arthroscopy of the elbow. *Clinics in Sports Medicine, 5*, 653.

Andrews, J.R., & Timmerman, L.A. (1995). Outcome of elbow surgery in professional baseball players. *American Journal of Sports Medicine, 23,* 407-413.

Andrews, J.R., Wilk, K.E., Satterwhite, Y.E., & Tedder, J.L. (1993). Physical examination of the thrower's elbow. *Journal of Orthopaedic and Sports Physical Therapy, 6,* 296-304.

Apfelberg, D.B., & Larson, S.J. (1973). Dynamic anatomy of the ulnar nerve at the elbow. *Plastic Reconstructive Surgery, 51,* 76.

Arrigo, C.M., Wilk, K.E., & Andrews, J.R. (1994). Peak torque and maximum work repetition during isokinetic testing of the shoulder internal and external rotators. *Isokinetics and Exercise Science, 4,* 171-175.

Ballantyne, B.T., O'Hare, S.J., Paschall, J.L., Pavia-Smith, M.M., Pitz, A.M., Gillon, J.F., & Soderberg, G.L. (1993). Electromyographic activity of selected shoulder muscles in commonly used therapeutic exercises. *Physical Therapy, 73,* 668-682.

Barnes, D.A., & Tullos, H.S. (1978). An analysis of 100 symptomatic baseball players. *American Journal of Sports Medicine, 6,* 62-67.

Barrentine, S.W. (1994, January). *Biomechanics of underhand softball pitching.* Paper presented at the 12th Annual Injuries in Baseball Course, Birmingham, AL.

Bennett, G.E. (1959). Elbow and shoulder lesions of baseball players. *American Journal of Surgery, 98,* 484-492.

Bennett, J.B., Green, M.S., & Tullos, H.S. (1992, May). Surgical management of chronic medial elbow instability. *Clinical Orthopaedics and Related Research, 278,* 62-68.

Bernhang, A.M., Dehner, W., & Fogarty, C. (1974). Tennis elbow: A biomechanical approach. *American Journal of Sports Medicine, 2,* 235-260.

Blackburn, T.A., McLeod, W.D., White, B., Wofford, L. (1990, Spring). EMG analysis of posterior rotator cuff exercises. *Athletic Training, 25,* 40-45.

Bonutti, P.M., Windau, J.E., Ables, B.A., & Miller, B.G. (1994). Static progressive stretch to reestablish elbow range of motion. *Clinical Orthopaedics and Related Research, 303,* 128-134.

Bowling, R.W., & Rockar, P.A. (1985). The elbow complex. In G.J. Davies & J.A. Gould (Eds.), *Orthopaedic and sports physical therapy* (pp. 476-496). St. Louis: Mosby.

Boyd, H.B., & Mcleod, A.C. (1973). Tennis elbow. *Journal of Bone and Joint Surgery, 55A*(6), 1183-1187.

Brattberg, G. (1983). Acupuncture therapy for tennis elbow. *Pain, 16,* 285-288.

Brody, H. (1989). Vibration dampening of tennis rackets. *International Journal of Sport Biomechanics, 5,* 451-456.

Butler, D.S. (1994). The upper limb tension test revisited. In R. Grant (Ed.), *Physical therapy of the cervical and thoracic spine* (pp. 217-244). New York: Churchill Livingston.

Carlson, J.S., & Cera, M.A. (1984, December). Cardiorespiratory, muscular strength and anthropometric characteristics of elite Australian junior male and female tennis players. *The Australian Journal of Science and Medicine in Sport, 16,* 7-13.

Carroll, R. (1981). Tennis elbow: Incidence in local league players. *British Journal of Sports Medicine, 15,* 250-255.

Chandler, T.J., Kibler, W.B., Stracener, E.C., Ziegler, A.K., Pace, B. (1992). Shoulder strength, power, and endurance in college tennis players. *American Journal of Sports Medicine, 20,* 455-458.

Chase, A.A., & Baker, C.L. (1994). Rehabilitation after elbow arthroscopy. *Orthopaedic Physical Therapy Clinics of North America, 3,* 507-524.

Chinn, C.J., Priest, J.D., & Kent, B.E. (1974). Upper extremity range of motion, grip strength, and girth in highly skilled tennis players. *Physical Therapy, 54,* 474-482.

Chu, D. (1989). *Plyometric exercises with the medicine ball.* Livermore, CA: Bittersweet.

Clancy, W.G. (1994, January). *Knee injuries in baseball.* Presented at the 12th Annual Injuries in Baseball Course, Birmingham, AL.

Cohen, D.B., Mont, M.A., Campbell, K.R., Vogelstein, B.N., & Loewy, J.W. (1994). Upper extremity physical factors affecting tennis serve velocity. *American Journal of Sports Medicine, 22,* 746-750.

Conway, J.E., Jobe, F.W., Glousman, R.E., & Pink, M. (1992). Medial instability of the elbow in throwing athletes. *The Journal of Bone and Joint Surgery, 74A*(1), 67-83.

Coonrad, R.W., Hooper, W.R. (1973). Tennis elbow. Its course, natural history, conservative and surgical management. *Journal of Bone and Joint Surgery, 55A*(6), 1177-1182.

Cooper, J.E., Shwedyk, E., Quanbury, A.O., Miller, J., & Hildebrand, D. (1993). Elbow joint restriction: Effect on functional upper limb motion during performance of three feeding activities. *Archives of Physical Medicine and Rehabilitation, 74,* 805-809.

Cybex, Incorporated. (1992). *Isolated joint testing and exercise.* Ronkonkoma, NY: Author.

Cyriax, J.H., & Cyriax, P.J. (1983). *Illustrated manual of orthopaedic medicine.* London: Butterworths.

Daniels, L., & Worthingham, C. (1980). *Muscle testing: Techniques of manual examination* (4th ed.). Philadelphia: W.B. Saunders.

Davidson, P.A., Pink, M., Perry, J., Jobe, F.W. (1995). Functional anatomy of the flexor pronator muscle group in relation to the medial collateral ligament of the elbow. *American Journal of Sports Medicine, 23*(2), 245-250.

Davies, G.J. (1985). *A compendium of isokinetics in clinical usage* (2nd ed.). LaCrosse, WI: S & S Publishers.

Davies, G.J. (1992). *A compendium of isokinetics in clinical usage* (4th ed.). LaCrosse, WI: S & S Publishers.

Davies, G.J., & Ellenbecker, T.S. (1992). Eccentric isokinetics. *Orthopaedic Physical Therapy Clinics of North America, 1*(2), 297-336.

Dijs, H., Mortier, G., Driessens, M., DeRidder, A., Willems, J., & Devroey, T. (1990). A retrospective study of the conservative treatment of tennis elbow. *Medica Physica, 13,* 73-77.

Dillman, C.J. (1991). *The upper extremity in tennis and throwing athletes.* Paper presented at the United States Tennis Association National Meeting, Tucson, AZ.

Dilorenzo, C.E., Parkes, J.C., & Chmelar, R.D. (1990). The importance of shoulder and cervical dysfunction in the etiology and treatment of athletic elbow injuries. *Journal of Orthopaedic and Sports Physical Therapy, 11,* 402-409.

Donkers, M.J., An, K.N., Chao, E.Y., & Morrey, B.F. (1993). Hand position affects elbow joint load during push-up exercise. *Journal of Biomechanics, 26,* 625-632.

Doss, W.S., & Karpovich, P.V. (1965). A comparison of concentric, eccentric, and isometric strength of the elbow flexors. *Journal of Applied Physiology, 20,* 351-353.

Ellenbecker, T.S. (1991). A total arm strength isokinetic profile of highly skilled tennis players. *Isokinetics and Exercise Science, 1*(1), 9-21.

Ellenbecker, T.S. (1992a). Elbow, forearm, and wrist testing and rehabilitation. In G.J. Davies (Ed.), *A compendium of isokinetics in clinical usage* (4th ed.) (pp. 481-496). LaCrosse, WI: S & S Publishers.

Ellenbecker, T.S. (1992b). Shoulder internal and external rotation strength and range of motion of highly skilled junior tennis players. *Isokinetics and Exercise Science, 2*(2), 1-8.

Ellenbecker, T.S. (1993, January). *Isokinetic muscular performance of the baseball pitcher.* Paper presented at the 11th Annual Injuries in Baseball Course, Birmingham, AL.

Ellenbecker, T.S. (1995). Rehabilitation of shoulder and elbow injuries in tennis players. *Clinics in Sports Medicine, 14*(1), 87-110.

Ellenbecker, T.S., Davies, G.J., & Rowinski, M.J. (1988). Concentric versus eccentric isokinetic strengthening of the rotator cuff: Objective data versus functional test. *American Journal of Sports Medicine, 16*(1), 64-69.

Ellenbecker, T.S., & Derscheid, G.L. (1989). Rehabilitation of overuse injuries of the shoulder. *Clinics in Sports Medicine, 8,* 583-604.

Ellenbecker, T.S., Kingma, J., & Kim, A. (1994). A six-week isotonic training study of the forearm flexors and extensors in healthy subjects (unpublished research).

Ellenbecker, T.S., & Roetert, E.P. (1994). Upper extremity range of motion of elite senior tennis players (unpublished data).

Esch, J.C., & Baker, C.L. (1993). *Arthroscopic surgery: The shoulder and elbow.* Philadelphia: J.P. Lippincott.

Feltner, M., & Dapena, J. (1986). Dynamics of the shoulder and elbow joints of the throwing arm during a baseball pitch. *International Journal of Sport Biomechanics, 2*, 235-259.

Fish, D.R., & Wingate, L. (1985). Sources of goniometric error at the elbow. *Physical Therapy, 65*, 1666-1670.

Fleck, S.J., & Kraemer, W.J. (1987). *Designing resistance training programs.* Champaign, IL: Human Kinetics.

Fleisig, G.S., & Barrentine, S.W. (1995). Biomechanical aspects of the elbow in sports. *Sports Medicine and Arthroscopy Review, 3*, 149-159.

Fleisig, G.S., Dillman, C.J., & Andrews, J.R. (1989). Proper mechanics for baseball pitching. *Clinical Sports Medicine, 1*, 151-170.

Francis, K., & Hoobler, T. (1986). Comparison of peak torque values of the knee flexor and extensor muscle groups using the Cybex II and Lido 2.0 isokinetic dynamometers. *Journal of Orthopaedic and Sports Physical Therapy, 8*, 480-483.

Froimson, A.I. (1971). Treatment of tennis elbow with forearm support band. *Journal of Bone and Joint Surgery, 53A*, 183-184.

Galloway, M., DeMaio, M., & Mangine, R. (1992). Rehabilitative techniques in the treatment of medial and lateral epicondylitis. *Sports Medicine Rehabilitation Series, 15*, 1089-1096.

Garden, R.S. (1961). Tennis elbow. *Journal of Bone and Joint Surgery, 43B*, 100.

Giangarra, C.E., Conroy, B., Jobe, F.W., Pink, M., & Perry, J. (1993). Electromyographic and cinematographic analysis of elbow function in tennis players using single- and double-handed backhand strokes. *American Journal of Sports Medicine, 21*(3), 394-399.

Glazebrook, M.A., Curwin, S., Islam, M.N., Kozey, J., & Stanish, W.D. (1994). *American Journal of Sports Medicine, 22*, 674-679.

Glousman, R.E., Barron, J., Jobe, F.W., Perry, J., & Pink, M. (1992). An electromyographic analysis of the elbow in normal and injured pitchers with medial collateral ligament insufficiency. *American Journal of Sports Medicine, 20*(3), 311-317.

Goitz, H.T., Rijke, A.M., Andrews, J.R., Phillips, B.B., & McCue, F.C. (1994). Elbow ulnar collateral ligament disruption: A new, non-invasive diagnostic technique (Abstract). Presented at February 1993 AOSSM Society Specialty Day Meeting, San Francisco.

Goldie, I. (1964). Epicondylitis lateralis humeri. *Acta Chir. Scand. Suppl., 339*, 1-114.

Gould, J.A., & Davies, G.J. (1985). Orthopaedic and sports rehabilitation concepts. In J.A. Gould & G.J. Davies (Eds.), *Orthopaedic and sports physical therapy* (pp. 181-198). St. Louis: Mosby.

Grabiner, M.D., Groppel, J.L., Campbell, K.R. (1983). Resultant tennis ball velocity as a function of off-center impact and grip firmness. *Medicine and Science in Sports and Exercise, 15*, 542-544.

Graviss, E.R., & Hoffman, A.D. (1993). Imaging of the pediatric elbow. In B.F. Morrey (Ed.), *The elbow and its disorders* (2nd ed.) (pp. 181-188). Philadelphia: W.B. Saunders.

Groppel, J.L. (1992). *High tech tennis* (2nd ed.). Champaign, IL: Human Kinetics.

Groppel, J.L., & Nirschl, R.P. (1986). A biomechanical and electromyographical analysis of the effects of counterforce braces on the tennis player. *American Journal of Sports Medicine, 14*(3), 195-200.

Halls, A.A., & Travill, A. (1964). Transmission of pressures across the elbow joint. *Anat. Rec, 150,* 243-248.

Hanavan, E.P. (1964). *A mathematical model of the human body.* (Contract No. AMRL-TR-64-102). Dayton, OH: Wright-Patterson Air Force Base.

Hang, Y.S., & Peng, S.M. (1984). An epidemiological study of upper extremity injury in tennis players with particular reference to tennis elbow. *Journal of the Formosan Medical Association, 83,* 307-316.

Hawkins, R.J., & Kennedy, J. (1980). Impingement syndrome in athletes. *American Journal of Sports Medicine, 8,* 151-158.

Henry, A.K. (1957). *Extensive exposure* (2nd ed.). Baltimore: Williams & Wilkins.

Hepburn, G.R., & Crivelli, K.J. (1984). Use of elbow dynasplint for reduction of elbow flexion contractures: A case study. *Journal of Orthopaedic and Sports Physical Therapy, 5,* 269-274.

Heyse-Moore, G.H. (1984). Resistant tennis elbow. *Journal of Hand Surgery, 9,* 64-66.

Hodges, C. (1992). The upper limb tension test in competitive baseball pitchers. Unpublished master's thesis, School of Physiotherapy, University of South Australia.

Hoppenfeld, S. (1976). *Physical examination of the spine and extremities.* Norwalk, CT: Appleton-Century-Crofts (Prentice-Hall).

Huddleston, A.L., Rockwell, D., Kulund, D.N., & Harrison, B. (1980). Bone mass in lifetime tennis athletes. *Journal of the American Medical Association, 244,* 1107-1109.

Ilfeld, F.W. (1992). Can stroke modification relieve tennis elbow? *Clinical Orthopaedics and Related Research, 276,* 182-186.

Indelicato, P.A., Jobe, F.W., Kerlan, R.K., Carter, V.S., Shields, C.L., & Lombardo, S.J. (1979). Correctable elbow lesions in professional baseball players: A review of 25 cases. *American Journal of Sports Medicine, 7,* 72-75.

Ingham, (1981). Transverse cross friction massage. *The Physician and Sports Medicine, 9*(10), 116.

Inglis, A.E. (1991). The rehabilitation of the elbow after injury. In H.S. Tullos (Ed.), *Instructional Course Lectures, XL,* 45-49.

Jobe, F.W., & Elattrache, N.S. (1993). Diagnosis and treatment of ulnar collateral ligament injuries in athletes. In B.F. Morrey (Ed.), *The elbow and its disorders* (2nd ed.) (pp. 566-572). Philadelphia: W.B. Saunders.

Jobe, F.W., Fanton, G.S., & Elattrache, N.S. (1993). Ulnar nerve injury. In B.F. Morrey (Ed.), *The elbow and its disorders* (2nd ed.) (pp. 560-565): Philadelphia: W.B. Saunders.

Jobe, F.W., & Kvitne, R.S. (1989) Shoulder pain in the overhand or throwing athlete: The relationship of anterior instability and rotator cuff impingement. *Orthopaedic Review, 28*(9), 963-975.

Jobe, F.W., & Kvitne, R.S. (1991). Elbow instability in the athlete. In. H.S. Tullos (Ed.), *Instructional Course Lectures, XL,* 17-23.

Jobe, F.W., Moynes, D.R., & Antonelli, D.J. (1986). Rotator cuff function during a golf swing. *American Journal of Sports Medicine, 14,* 388-392.

Jobe, F.W., Stark, H., & Lombardo, S.J. (1986). Reconstruction of the ulnar collateral ligament in athletes. *Journal of Bone and Joint Surgery, 68A,* 1158-1163.

Joyce, M.E., Jelsma, R.D., & Andrews, J.R. (1995). Throwing injuries to the elbow. *Sports Medicine and Arthroscopy Review, 3,* 224-236.

Kaltenborn, F.M. (1980). *Mobilization of the extremity joints* (3rd ed.). Oslo, Norway: Olaf Norlis.

Kamien, M. (1990). A rational management of tennis elbow. *Sports Medicine, 9,* 173-191.

Kannus, P. Maupasalo, H., Sankelo, M., Fievänen, H., Pasanen, M., Heinenen, A., Oja, P., Vueri, I. (1995). Effect of starting age of physical activity on bone mass on the dominant arm of tennis and squash players. *Anals of Internal Medicine, 123,* 27-31.

Kapandji, I.A. (1970). *The physiology of the joints.* London: Churchill Livingstone.

Kelley, J.D., Lombardo, S.J., Pink, M., Perry, J., & Giangarra, C.E. (1994). Electromyographic and cinematographic analysis of elbow function in tennis players with lateral epicondylitis. *American Journal of Sports Medicine, 22,* 359-363.

Kendall, F.D., & McCreary, E.K. (1983). *Muscle testing and function* (3rd ed.). Baltimore: Williams and Wilkins.

Kessler, R.M., & Hertling, D. (1983). *Management of common musculoskeletal disorders: Physical therapy principles and methods.* Philadelphia: Harper & Row.

Kibler, W.B. (1994). Clinical biomechanics of the elbow in tennis: Implications for evaluation and diagnosis. *Medicine and Science in Sports and Exercise, 26,* 1203-1206.

King, G.J.W., Morrey, B.F., & An, K.N. (1993). Stabilizers of the elbow. *Journal of Shoulder and Elbow Surgery, 2*(3), 165-174.

King, J.W., Brelsford, H.J., & Tullos, H.S. (1969). Analysis of the pitching arm of the professional baseball pitcher. *Clinical Orthopaedics, 67,* 116-123.

Kiriti, S., & Unthoff, H.K. (1980). Ultrastructure of the common extensor tendon in tennis elbow. *Virchows Arch, 386,* 317-330.

Kitai, E., Itay, S., Ruder, A., Engel, J., & Modan, M. (1986). An epidemiological study of lateral epicondylitis in amateur male players. *Ann. Chir. Main, 5,* 113-121.

Kivi, P. (1982). The etiology and conservative treatment of humeral epicondylitis. *Scandinavian Journal of Rehabilitative Medicine, 15,* 37-42.

Komi, P.V., & Buskirk, E.R. (1972). Quantitative evaluation of mechanical and electrical changes during fatigue loading of eccentric and concentric work. *Scandinavian Journal of Rehabilitative Medicine, 3*(Suppl.), 21-26.

Krahl, H., Michaelis, U., Pieper, H.G., Quack, G., & Montag, M. (1994). Stimulation of bone growth in the upper extremities in professional tennis players. *American Journal of Sports Medicine, 22,* 751-757.

Kuessner, U. (1991). Vibration dampeners: Do they work? *Tennis Australia, 16,* 57.

Kulund, D.N., Rockwell, D., & Brubaker, C.E. (1979). The long-term effects of playing tennis. *The Physician and Sportsmedicine, 7*(4), 87-92.

Kuroda, S., & Sakamaki, K. (1986). Ulnar collateral ligament tears of the elbow joint. *Clinical Orthopaedics and Related Research, 208,* 266-271.

Labelle, H., Guibert, R., Joncas, J., Newman, N., Fallaha, M., & Rivard, C.H. (1992). Lack of scientific evidence for the treatment of lateral epicondylitis of the elbow. *Journal of Bone and Joint Surgery, 74B,* 646-651.

Leadbetter, W.B. (1992). Cell matrix response in tendon injury. *Clinics in Sports Medicine, 11,* 533-579.

Loosli, A.R., Requa, R.K., Garrick, J.G., & Hanley, E. (1992). Injuries to pitchers in women's collegiate fast-pitch softball. *American Journal of Sports Medicine, 20*(1), 35-37.

Lynch, G.J., Meyers, J.F., Whipple, T.L., & Caspari, R.B. (1986). Anatomy and elbow arthroscopy: Inherent risks. *Arthroscopy, 2,* 191.

Magee, D.J. (1987). *Orthopedic physical assessment.* Philadelphia: Saunders.

Maitland, G.D. (1970). *Vertebral manipulation.* London: Butterworths.

Mawdsley, R.H., & Knapik, J.J. (1982). Comparison of isokinetic measurements with test repetitions. *Physical Therapy, 62,* 169.

Mero, A., Komi, T.V., Korjus, T., Navarro, E., Gregor, R.J. (1994). Body segment contributions to javelin throwing during final thrust phase. *Journal of Applied Biomechanics, 10,* 166-177.

Miyashita, M., Tsunoda, T., Sakurai, S., Nishizono, H., & Mizuno, T. (1980). Muscular activities in the tennis serve and overhand throwing. *Scandinavian Journal of Sports Science, 2*(2), 52-58.

Morrey, B.F. (1992a). Posttraumatic stiffness: Distraction arthroplasty. *Orthopaedics, 15,* 863-869.

Morrey, B.F. (1992b). Primary degenerative arthritis of the elbow: Treatment by ulnohumeral arthroplasty. *Journal of Bone and Joint Surgery, 74B,* 409-413.

Morrey, B.F. (Ed.) (1993). *The elbow and its disorders* (2nd ed.). Philadelphia: W.B. Saunders.

Morrey, B.F. (1994). *The Elbow*. In R.C. Thompson, Jr. Master Techniques in Orthopaedic Surgery Series. New York: Raven Press.

Morrey, B.F., & An, K.N. (1983). Articular and ligamentous contributions to the stability of the elbow joint. *American Journal of Sports Medicine, 11,* 315.

Morrey, B.F., Askew, L.J., An, K.N, & Chao, E.Y. (1981). A biomechanical study of normal functional elbow motion. *Journal of Bone and Joint Surgery, 63A,* 872-877.

Morris, M., Jobe, F.W., Perry, J., Pink, M., & Healy, B.S. (1989). Electromyographic analysis of elbow function in tennis players. *American Journal of Sports Medicine, 17,* 241-247.

Moseley, V.B., Jobe, F.W., Pink, M., Perry, J., & Tibone, J. (1992). EMG analysis of the scapular muscles during a shoulder rehabilitation program. *American Journal of Sports Medicine, 20*(2), 128-134.

Neer, C.S. (1983). Impingement lesions. *Clinical Orthopaedics, 173,* 70-77.

Nirschl, R.P. (1977). Tennis elbow. *Primary Care, 4,* 367-382.

Nirschl, R.P. (1984). Tennis elbow: Joint resolution by conservative treatment and improved technique. *The Physician and Sportsmedicine, 12,* 168-182.

Nirschl, R.P. (1992). Elbow tendinosis/tennis elbow. *Clinics in Sports Medicine, 11,* 851-870.

Nirschl, R.P. (1993). In B.F. Morrey (Ed.), *The elbow and its disorders* (2nd ed.) (pp. 537-552). Philadelphia: W.B. Saunders.

Nirschl, R.P., & Sobel, J. (1981). Conservative treatment of tennis elbow. *The Physician and Sportsmedicine, 9*(6), 43-54.

Noyes, F.R., Mangine, R.E., & Barber, S.E. (1987). Early knee motion after open and arthroscopic anterior cruciate ligament reconstruction. *American Journal of Sports Medicine, 15,* 149-160.

O'Driscoll, S.W., Bell, D.F., & Morrey, B.F. (1991). Posterolateral rotary instability of the elbow. *Journal of Bone and Joint Surgery, 74A,* 440-446.

O'Driscoll, S.W., & Morrey, B.F. (1992). Arthroscopy of the elbow. *Journal of Bone and Joint Surgery, 72A*(1), 84-94.

Oglivie-Harris, D.J., Gordon, R., & MacKay, M. (1995). Arthroscopic treatment for posterior impingement in degenerative arthritis of the elbow. *Arthroscopy: The Journal of Arthroscopic and Related Surgery, 11,* 437-443.

Ollivierre, C.O., Nirschl, R.P., & Pettrone, F.A. (1995). Resection and repair for medial tennis elbow. A prospective analysis. *American Journal of Sports Medicine 23*(2): 214-221.

Palmitier, R.A., An, K.A., Scott, S.G., & Chao, E.Y.S. (1991). Kinetic chain exercise in knee rehabilitation. *Sports Medicine, 11,* 402-413.

Pechan & Julius (1975). Pressure measurement in the ulnar nerve: A contribution to the pathophysiology of the carpal tunnel syndrome. *Journal of Biomechanics, 8*(1), 75-79.

Percy, E.C., & Carson, J.D. (1981). The use of DMSO in tennis elbow and rotator cuff tendinitis: A double blind study. *Medicine and Science in Sports and Exercise, 13*, 215-219.

Perry, J., & Glousman, R. (1990). Biomechanics of throwing. In J.A. Nicholas & E.B. Hershman (Eds.), *The upper extremity in sports medicine* (pp. 727-750). St. Louis: Mosby.

Priest, J.D., Braden, V., & Gerberich, S.G. (1980). The elbow and tennis (Part 1): An analysis of players with and without pain. *The Physician and Sports Medicine, 8*(4), 81-91.

Priest, J.D., Jones, H.H., & Nagel, D.A. (1974). Elbow injuries in highly skilled tennis players. *Journal of Sports Medicine, 2*(3), 137-149.

Priest, J.D., Jones, H.H., Tichenor, C.J.C., et al. (1977). Arm and elbow changes in expert tennis players. *Minnesota Medicine, 60*, 399-404.

Priest, J.D., & Nagel, D.A. (1976). Tennis shoulder. *American Journal of Sports Medicine, 4*, 28-42.

Rang, M. (1983). *Children's fractures* (2nd ed.). Philadelphia: J.B. Lippincott.

Regan, W.D., Korinek, S.L., Morrey, B.F., & An, K.N. (1991). Biomechanical study of ligaments around the elbow joint. *Clinical Orthopaedics, 271*, 170-179.

Rettig, A.C., & Ebben, J.R. (1993). Anterior subcutaneous transfer of the ulnar nerve in the athlete. *American Journal of Sports Medicine, 21*, 836-840.

Rhu, K.N., McCormick, J., Jobe, F.W., et al. (1988). An electromyographic analysis of shoulder function in tennis players. *American Journal of Sports Medicine, 16*, 481-485.

Roetert, E.P., Brody, H., Dillman, C.J., Groppel, J.L., & Schultheis, J.M. (1995). *Clinics in Sports Medicine, 14*(1), 47-58.

Roles, N.C., & Mawdsley, R.H. (1972). Radial tunnel syndrome. *Journal of Bone and Joint Disorders, 54B*, 499-508.

Rosenthal, M. (1984). The efficacy of flurbiprofen versus piroxicam in the treatment of acute soft tissue rheumatism. *Current Medical Research and Opinion, 9*, 304-309.

Runge, F. (1873). Zur genese unt behand lung bes schreibekramp fes, *Berl Kun Woschenschr, 10*, 245.

Sakurai, S., Ikegami, Y., Okamoto, A., Yabe, K., & Toyoshima, S. (1993). A three- dimensional cinematographic analysis of upper limb movement during fastball and curveball baseball pitches. *Journal of Applied Biomechanics, 9*(1), 47-65.

Salter, R.B., & Harris, W.R. (1963). Injuries involving the epiphyseal plate. *Journal of Bone and Joint Surgery, 45A*, 587-X.

Salter, R.B., Simmonds, D.F., Malcolm, B.W., Rumble, E.J., MacMicheal, D., & Clements, N. (1980). The effects of continuous passive motion on healing of full thickness defects in articular cartilage. *Journal of Bone and Joint Surgery, 62A*, 1232-1251.

Schmier, A.A. (1945). Research work on a more precise method of determining muscle strength in poliomyelitis patients. *Journal of Bone and Joint Surgery, 27*, 317-326.

Seiler, J.G., Parker, L.M., Chamberland, P.D., Sherbourne, G.M., Carpenter, W.A. (1995). The Distal Biceps Tendon. *Journal of Shoulder and Elbow Surgery, 4*(3), 149-156.

Selvaratnam, P.J., Matyas, T.A., & Glasgow, E.F. (1994). Noninvasive discrimination of brachial plexus involvement in upper limb pain. *Spine, 19*(1), 26-33.

Seto, J.L., Brewster, C.E., Randall, C.C., & Jobe, F.W. (1991). *Journal of Orthopaedic and Sports Physical Therapy, 14*(3), 100-105.

Sisto, D., et al. (1987). An electromyographic analysis of the elbow in pitching. *American Journal of Sports Medicine, 15*(3), 260-263.

Slocum, D.B. (1978). Classification of the elbow injuries from baseball pitching. *American Journal of Sports Medicine, 6*, 62.

Smith, R., & Brunolli, J. (1989). Shoulder kinesthesia after anterior glenohumeral dislocation. *Physical Therapy, 69*(2), 106-112.

Snyder-Mackler, L., & Epler, M. (1989). Effects of standard and Aircast tennis elbow bands on integrated electromyography of forearm extensor musculature proximal to the bands. *American Journal of Sports Medicine, 17*, 278-281.

Sojbjerg, J.O., Ovesen, J., & Nielsen, S. (1987). Experimental elbow instability after transection of the medial collateral ligament. *Clinical Orthopaedics and Related Research, 218*, 186-190.

Sölveborn, S.A., & Olerud, C. (1996). Radial epicondylalgia (tennis elbow): Measurement of range of motion of the wrist and elbow. *Journal of Orthopaedic and Sports Physical Therapy, 23*(4), 251-257.

Sprigings, E., Marshall, R., Elliott, B., & Jennings, L. (1994). A three-dimensional kinematic method for determining the effectiveness of arm segment rotations in producing racquet-head speed. *Journal of Biomechanics, 27*, 245-254.

Stonecipher, D.R., & Catlin, P.A. (1984). The effect of a forearm strap on wrist extensor strength. *Journal of Orthopaedic and Sports Physical Therapy, 6*, 184-189.

Stovall, P.B., & Bernfield, M.S. (1979). Treatment of resistant lateral epicondylitis of the elbow by lengthening of the extensor carpi radialis brevis tendon. *Surg. Gynecol. Obstet., 149*, 526.

Stratford, P.W., Levy, D.R., Gauldie, S., Miseferi, D., Levy, K. (1989). The evaluation of phonophoresis and friction massage as treatments for extensor carpi radialis tendinitis: a randomized controlled trial. *Physiotherapy Canada, 41*, 93-99.

Strizak, A.M., Gleim, G.W., Sapega, A., & Nicholas, J.M. (1983). Hand and forearm strength and its relation to tennis. *American Journal of Sports Medicine, 11*, 234-239.

Stroyan, M., & Wilk, K.E. (1993). The functional anatomy of the elbow complex. *Journal of Orthopaedic and Sports Physical Therapy, 17*, 279-288.

Sullivan, P.E., Markos, P.D., & Minor, M.D. (1982). *An integrated approach to therapeutic exercise: Theory and clinical application.* Reston, VA: Reston.

Timmerman, L.A., & Andrews, J.R. (1994a). Clinical experience. In J.R. Andrews & S.R. Soffer (Eds.), *Elbow arthroscopy* (pp. 131-139). St. Louis: Mosby.

Timmerman, L.A., & Andrews, J.R. (1994b). Histology and arthroscopic anatomy of the ulnar collateral ligament of the elbow. *American Journal of Sports Medicine, 22*, 667-673.

Timmerman, L.A., & Andrews, J.R. (1994c). Undersurface tear of the ulnar collateral ligament in baseball players. *American Journal of Sports Medicine, 22*(1), 33-36.

Timmerman, L.A., Schwartz, M.L., & Andrews, J.R. (1994). Preoperative evaluation of the ulnar collateral ligament by magnetic resonance imaging and computed tomography arthrography: Evaluation in 25 baseball players with surgical confirmation. *American Journal of Sports Medicine, 22*(1), 26-32.

Torg, J.S., Pollack, H., Swetersitsch, P. (1972). The effect of competitive pitching on the preadolescent baseball player. *Pediatrics, 49*, 267-272.

Townsend, H., Jobe, F.W., Pink, M., & Perry, J. (1991). Electromyographic analysis of the glenohumeral muscles during a baseball rehabilitation program. *American Journal of Sports Medicine, 19*(3), 264-272.

Tullos, H.S., & King, J.W. (1973). Throwing mechanism in sports. *Orthopaedic Clinics in North America, 4*, 709-721.

VanGheluwe, B., & Hebbelinck, M. (1986). Muscle actions and ground reaction forces in tennis. *International Journal of Sport Biomechanics, 2*, 88-99.

Vanswearingen, J.W. (1983). Measuring wrist muscle strength. *Journal of Orthopaedic and Sports Physical Therapy, 4*, 217-228.

Vodak, P.A., Savin, W.M., & Haskell, W.L. (1980). Physiological profile of middle-aged male and female tennis players. *Medicine and Science in Sports and Exercise, 12*, 159-163.

Wadsworth, T.G. (1987). Tennis elbow: Conservative, surgical, and manipulative treatment. *British Medical Journal, 294*, 621-624.

Warner, J.J.P, Micheli, L.J, Arslanian, L.E., Kennedy, J., & Kennedy, R. (1990). Patterns of flexibility, laxity, and strength in normal shoulders and shoulders with instability and impingement. *American Journal of Sports Medicine, 18*, 366-375.

Werner, F.W., & An, K.N. (1994). Biomechanics of the elbow and forearm. *Hand Clin, 10*, 357-373.

Werner, S.L., Fleisig, G.S., Dillman, C.J., & Andrews, J.A. (1993). Biomechanics of the elbow during baseball pitching. *Journal of Orthopaedic and Sports Physical Therapy, 17*, 274-278.

Whiteside, J.A., & Andrews, J.R. (1995). Tendinopathies of the elbow. *Sports Medicine and Arthroscopy Review, 3,* 195-203.

Wilhite, M.R., Cohen, E.R., & Wilhite, S.C. (1992). Reliability of concentric and eccentric isokinetic movements: The effects of testing order for three different speeds. *Journal of Orthopaedic and Sports Physical Therapy, 15*(4), 175-182.

Wilk, K.E., & Arrigo, C.A. (1993). Current concepts in the rehabilitation of the athletic shoulder. *Journal of Orthopaedic and Sports Physical Therapy, 18,* 365-378.

Wilk, K.E., Arrigo, C.A., & Andrews, J.A. (1991). Standardized isokinetic testing protocol for the throwing shoulder. *Isokinetics and Exercise Science, 1*(2), 63-71.

Wilk, K.E., Arrigo, C.A., & Andrews, J.R. (1993). Rehabilitation of the elbow in the throwing athlete. *Journal of Orthopaedic and Sports Physical Therapy, 17,* 305-317.

Wilk, K.E., Azar, F.M., & Andrews, J.R. (1995). Conservative and operative rehabilitation of the elbow in sports. *Sports Medicine and Arthroscopy Review, 3,* 237-258.

Wilson, F.D., Andrews, J.A., Blackburn, T.A., & McCluskey, G. (1983). Valgus extension overload in the pitching elbow. *American Journal of Sports Medicine, 11*(2), 83-88.

Winge, S., Jorgensen, U., & Nielsen, A.L. (1989). Epidemiology of injuries in Danish championship tennis. *International Journal of Sports Medicine, 10,* 368-371.

Yoshizawa, M., Itani, T., & Jonsson, B. (1987). Muscular load in shoulder and forearm muscles in tennis players with different levels of skill. In B. Jonsson (Ed.), *Biomechanics X-B* (pp. 621-627). Champaign, IL: Human Kinetics.

Zachazewski, J.E., & Reischl, S. (1986). Flexibility for the runner: Specific program considerations. *Topics in Acute Care and Trauma Rehabilitation, 1,* 9-27.

Index

About the Authors

Todd Ellenbecker, MS, PT, SCS, CSCS, is the clinic director at the Physiotherapy Associates Sports Clinic in Scottsdale, Arizona. He is certified by the American Physical Therapy Association (APTA) as a sports clinical specialist, one of a limited number in the United States. This distinction requires five years of sports medicine experience and successful completion of an extensive written exam. He has treated elbow injuries in many professional baseball players and elite tennis players, having worked with the Milwaukee Brewers, Oakland A's, San Francisco Giants, and the United States Tennis Association.

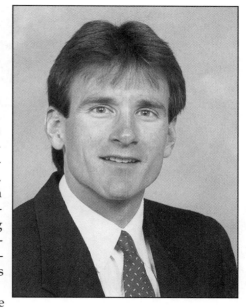

A member of the APTA and the American College of Sports Medicine, Ellenbecker has published many articles and research studies pertaining to the upper extremity in baseball and tennis players. He earned a bachelor's degree in physical therapy from the University of Wisconsin-LaCrosse and a master's degree in exercise physiology from Arizona State University.

Angelo J. Mattalino, MD, is an orthopaedic surgeon with Southwest Sports Medicine and Orthopaedic Surgery Clinic in Scottsdale, Arizona. He is an orthopaedic consultant to several professional baseball teams and the medical director of Major League Baseball's Arizona Fall League. He also works with the United States rugby, ski, and soccer teams; the Association of Tennis Professionals; and numerous high school teams.

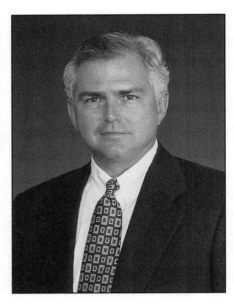

Dr. Mattalino, who earned a medical degree from the University of Texas, is certified by the American Board of Orthopaedic Surgeons and the Arthroscopy Board of North America. Following his orthopaedic surgical residency at Tulane Medical School, he completed fellowships in sports injuries and arthroscopy.

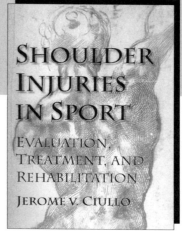
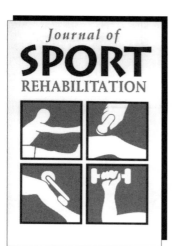